Praise for *The New Menopause Kitchen*

"*The New Menopause Kitchen* is full of practical information and an easy-to-follow plan that will be life-changing for millions of women. This is a MUST-read!"

—Sheinelle Jones, cohost of *The Today Show*
and *Today with Jenna & Sheinelle*
and author of *Through Mom's Eyes*

"Dr. Ian has been helping millions of Americans for years with his awesome, easily accessible plans. *The New Menopause Kitchen* continues that tradition and will help millions of women in this transformative period of their life and beyond."

—Rachael Ray, Emmy Award–winning TV host,
#1 *New York Times* bestselling author,
and internationally acclaimed cook

"*The New Menopause Kitchen* offers millions of women a chance to harness the natural power of nutrition to help address the symptoms of menopause, food first. This is a much-needed game changer!"

—Dr. Jennifer Ashton, founder of Ajenda and
board-certified OB-GYN and nutritionist

"Dr. Ian Smith, the trusted authority who's empowered millions through 30 books, most of them bestsellers, and national health initiatives, delivers again with *The New Menopause Kitchen*. Grounded in robust science and his decades of expertise, this gem offers Rachael Ray's delicious, menopause-thriving recipes to ease symptoms, melt stubborn weight, and reclaim vitality. A must-read for women navigating perimenopause, menopause, and beyond!"

—Barbara Hannah Grufferman, host of the *Age Better* podcast,
AARP columnist, and author of *Love Your Age*
and *The Best of Everything After 50*

The *NEW* Menopause Kitchen

Also by Ian K. Smith, MD

The Last 15
Eat Your Age
The Met Flex Diet
Plant Power
Burn Melt Shred
Fast Burn
Mind Over Weight
Clean & Lean
The Clean 20
Blast the Sugar Out!
The Shred Power Cleanse
The Shred Diet Cookbook
Super Shred
Shred
The Truth About Men
Eat
Happy
The 4 Day Diet
Extreme Fat Smash Diet
The Fat Smash Diet
The Take Control Diet
Dr. Ian's Guide to Medical Websites

Novels

Beyond Midnight: An Ashe Cayne Novel
Eagle Rock: An Ashe Cayne Novel
The Overnights: An Ashe Cayne Novel
Wolf Point: An Ashe Cayne Novel
The Unspoken: An Ashe Cayne Novel
The Ancient Nine
The Blackbird Papers

The *NEW* Menopause Kitchen

Targeted Nutrition to Help Fight Symptoms, Lose Weight, and Thrive in Perimenopause, Menopause, and Beyond

IAN K. SMITH, MD

BENBELLA
BenBella Books, Inc.
Dallas, TX

BenBella

BenBella Books, Inc.
8080 N. Central Expressway
Suite 1700
Dallas, TX 75206
benbellabooks.com
Send feedback to feedback@benbellabooks.com

BenBella is a federally registered trademark.

Printed in the United States of America
10 9 8 7 6 5 4 3 2 1

Library of Congress Control Number: 2026016057
ISBN 9781637749500 (hardcover)
ISBN 9781637749517 (electronic)

Editing by Leah Wilson and Karen Wise
Copyediting by Natalie Roth
Proofreading by Mary White and Lisa Story
Indexing by Debra Bowman
Text design and composition by Jordan Koluch
Cover design by Sarah Avinger
Cover image © Adobe Stock / stokkete
Printed by Lake Book Manufacturing

To my wife, Tristé, who is as beautiful, fearless,
and amazing as the first day we met crossing that famous avenue.
Thanks for always reminding me of my strength
and my ability to dream and achieve. What a ride!

Contents

Author's Note

For more than twenty years I have helped people around the world lose weight and improve their wellness. Most of my social media followers have been women who have engaged with me from one book to the next, fearlessly and confidently riding with me as I presented various plans with new, evolving science that showed different ways to reach wellness and fitness goals.

Several years ago, a close college friend asked me why I had never written a plan specifically for women who were about to go through menopause or who were in the midst of this seismic life change. I explained to her that I had written many plans, and many women facing this midlife change had found success with them. Why did I need to write a specific plan for menopause when women had found significant success with my other books?

To her credit, my friend not only pushed back but was relentless and kept the pressure on through the years. She explained that menopause presented a unique set of challenges that needed to be addressed with focus and special consideration. She made it clear that there were millions of women in need of not any old plan but one that spoke directly to them, a plan that would be sensitive to their specific needs and help them navigate this often-frustrating period of their life without judgment or shame.

A few years later, I was on a weekly Zoom call with a large group of women in one of my wellness Facebook groups when one of the women started talking about how she was in menopause and how everything had just seemed to slow down. No matter what she tried, she said, nothing was working to get the weight off and the bloat down, or counteract the other changes that were wreaking havoc on her life. She desperately needed something that would help her. I immediately heard my friend Peri's words in the back of my head and smiled. I asked the group if they thought a plan specifically addressing menopause would be helpful. The unified response was DEAFENING. "Absolutely! Of course! We need it NOW!" Several women even playfully chided me for not having written the plan already.

I listened to the feedback from these women (and finally Peri) and went about the work of researching menopause and everything associated with it. I found a treasure trove of extremely useful information—scientific studies, articles, opinion pieces, first-person accounts. There was so much to digest, and it wasn't only about the physical and physiological changes but also the psychological and psychosocial aspects involved with this transition. I grew even more excited when I discovered that while there were plenty of books written about perimenopause and menopause, there were less than a handful of books that focused on the interaction of menopause and food. There were even fewer books that actually offered women a specific plan that would assist them with weight loss and help diminish the frequency and impact of other common symptoms such as hot flashes, disrupted sleep, lowered energy levels, irritability, and anxiety.

I used all the research I discovered and the feedback from thousands of women and wrote *The New Menopause Kitchen*. I wanted not only to provide some real answers but to empower women so they could have more control over this period of their life. I wanted women to know that menopause was not an end, but the beginning of something new, exciting, and powerful, and that food—something we all love and cherish—could play a critical role in helping to provide the solutions they so desperately sought. While food was the centerpiece of the program, I also wanted to emphasize exercise, because it has been shown to be especially beneficial during this period of a woman's life, and unfortunately, most advice given to women has focused on medications and supplements. Exercise/physical activity has largely been ignored.

After I wrote the earlier versions of the plan, I allowed hundreds of women to try it and give me feedback. I was excited by both the great results they obtained and the personal stories of how their mindset and perspective changed and how they felt like they had finally regained control. Now, the plan that helped them is yours. As a bonus, I enlisted my great friend Rachael Ray, a globally celebrated cook and true food magician, to help create recipes that are not only delicious, affordable, and accessible, but comforting and specifically designed to help in your journey as you not only navigate but totally own how you experience this life-changing period.

1

THE WHAT AND THE WHY OF MENOPAUSE

We make hundreds of thousands, if not millions, of trips in our life. Whether we are preparing to visit a destination halfway around the world or traveling to the local grocery store on the other side of town, we don't only think about our destination. We also think about how we're going to get there. We have a plan—whether it's complicated or simple—to help us arrive safely at our desired destination.

Menopause is another journey that is best traveled with a plan, and a good plan starts with good fundamentals. This first chapter is all about giving you a solid foundation of basic facts so that all the information that follows makes sense, and you have sufficient knowledge to understand many of the terms and concepts involved in your menopausal journey. Informed decisions are almost always better decisions, and the knowledge you get in this chapter is meant to help and guide the choices you ultimately make.

It's critical to establish right away that menopause is not a disease, a malfunction, or a sign of weakness. It is a natural, biological milestone—one that signals a significant transformation in a woman's life. It marks the end of reproductive capability and ushers in a new stage that can be as vibrant, healthy, and empowering as any other phase of life. Historically, menopause has been misunderstood or even stigmatized and often equated with decline. The language around menopause has caused women to feel shame and inadequacy, which is extremely unfortunate and totally off the mark. The good news is that modern medicine and evolving cultural narratives are redefining menopause. We now understand that, with proper support and understanding, instead of feeling weakened and helpless, women can be full of strength, self-awareness, and renewed vitality.

From a biological standpoint, menopause is a complex hormonal shift involving the gradual decline of ovarian function and a significant drop in the production of the hormones estrogen and progesterone. These hormonal changes impact nearly every system in the body—not just the reproductive organs often discussed. It's important for women and their healthcare providers to be cognizant of and responsive to these dramatic changes as they have both short- and long-term health consequences, many of which can be prevented or mitigated with appropriate interventions.

The numbers make menopause's significance clear: According to the US Census Bureau, more than 50 million women in the United States are currently in menopause or postmenopause, and that number is projected to grow substantially as life expectancy continues to rise. Globally, the World Health Organization estimates that by 2030, more than 1.2 billion women will be age fifty and older.[1] It's now become evident that with the average life expectancy for women now reaching into the eighties, many women will spend up to one-third of their lives in the postmenopausal stage.

It's critical to acknowledge and understand that menopause is not just a fleeting transition, rather it's a major life phase. In fact, studies show that nearly 75 percent of women experience moderate to severe menopausal symptoms that affect their quality of life, work productivity, and mental health. Vasomotor symptoms—such as hot flashes and night sweats—are reported by 60 percent to 80 percent of women and may persist for more than seven years. Despite the prevalence and impact of these symptoms, many women feel unprepared for menopause. In fact, in a 2025 study reported in the *Mayo Clinic Proceedings*, approximately 87 percent of women did not seek medical care for menopause symptoms, with most of them citing the reasons of "being too busy" or "lacking awareness about effective treatment options."[2] This is an old and negligent cycle that definitely needs to be broken. Thankfully, the times when women were not expected, allowed, or supported to talk about their menopausal experience are in the past, and open, honest, meaningful conversations can now be had without fear, shame, or retaliation. Like most situations in life, empowerment starts with education, and it is time we elevate the conversation around menopause to give women the knowledge, tools, and validation they deserve during this critical life transition.

Menopause unfolds in three distinct but interconnected stages: perimenopause, menopause, and postmenopause. Perimenopause is the beginning, the transition phase marked by irregular cycles and fluctuating hormones. This is when things start to change, and when many women begin to take notice of these changes. Actual menopause is officially diagnosed after a woman goes twelve consecutive months without menstruation. The symptoms women experience tend to be most severe and unpredictable during that year. The third stage is postmenopause, and as the name indicates, this period includes all the years after menopause. It's important to understand these distinct stages as each one presents its own set of physical and emotional changes that require different approaches to support and care.

The Three Stages of Menopause

Perimenopause	Menopause	Postmenopause
• Leads up to menopause • Symptoms begin for many women	• 12 months since last period • Symptoms fluctuate	• After menopause • Symptoms may ease

PERIMENOPAUSE

Perimenopause, often referred to as the menopausal transition, marks the beginning of the hormonal shifts that lead to menopause. This phase can begin in a woman's late thirties to early forties and may last anywhere from two to ten years. It is initiated when the ovaries begin to decline in function, leading to the irregular production of estrogen and progesterone, the key reproductive hormones. Unlike in the reproductive years, when hormones rise and fall in predictable patterns, hormone levels during perimenopause fluctuate unpredictably, and this contributes to the wide variety of symptoms and frustration experienced by many women.

During perimenopause, ovulation (the process in which a mature egg is released by the ovary where it can be picked up by the fallopian tube and also the time in the menstrual cycle when pregnancy is most likely to occur) becomes erratic, and menstrual cycles become increasingly irregular. A woman might go several months without a period and then experience a heavy or prolonged cycle. These inconsistencies can be confusing and sometimes concerning, especially when they are accompanied by other physical and emotional symptoms. Estrogen dominance, where estrogen temporarily outweighs progesterone, can occur at times and may intensify symptoms such as breast tenderness, bloating, and mood swings.

The hormonal unpredictability during this time often gives rise to symptoms such as: (1) hot flashes and night sweats; (2) irritability, anxiety, and mood swings; (3) fatigue and brain fog; (4) breast tenderness; (5) sleep disturbances; and (6) irregular periods. These symptoms may vary significantly in intensity and frequency from one woman to another. However, studies have shown that nearly 80 percent of women experience some form of vasomotor symptoms during perimenopause, and for many, these symptoms are more intense during perimenopause than during menopause itself.[3]

In addition to physical symptoms, emotional and cognitive changes are common. Fluctuating hormone levels impact neurotransmitters—chemical messengers—such as serotonin and dopamine, which are crucial for mood regulation. This can lead to increased emotional sensitivity, irritability, or a feeling of being overwhelmed. Women in this stage are often also juggling career demands, caregiving for children or aging parents, spousal/partner relationships, and other stressors, and these can amplify the psychological burden of these hormonal changes.

Understanding that these changes are part of a natural biological process can help normalize the experience and reduce fear or shame. Tracking symptoms and cycles can also provide valuable insights and help women prepare for the next stage—menopause itself. Healthcare providers may recommend lifestyle changes, hormone evaluations, or symptom-specific interventions to ease this transition and maintain well-being during this unpredictable phase.

MENOPAUSE

Menopause is diagnosed retrospectively and refers to the specific point in time when a woman has not had a menstrual period for twelve consecutive months. According to the Mayo Clinic, the average age of natural menopause in the United States is approximately fifty-one, though it may occur earlier due to genetic factors, lifestyle influences such as smoking, or medical causes such as oophorectomy (surgical removal of ovaries), chemotherapy, or pelvic radiation therapy. It's important to note that no two women experience menopause exactly the same way. While there can be lots of similarities, menopause is truly a unique experience.

This phase marks the permanent end of fertility and comes with a significant drop in estrogen and progesterone levels due to the end of ovarian follicular activity. As a result, women experience physiological shifts that can manifest in various physical and emotional symptoms. Some symptoms continue from perimenopause, while others may become more pronounced or now appear for the first time. Common symptoms during menopause include:

- **Vasomotor symptoms** such as hot flashes and night sweats, which can affect sleep and overall quality of life. Research from the Study of Women's Health Across the Nation (SWAN) indicates that over 75 percent of women experience vasomotor symptoms during menopause, and these may last for seven to eleven years after they are first experienced.[4]
- **Urogenital atrophy**, leading to vaginal dryness, pain during intercourse, and urinary tract discomfort. According to a 2026 article in *Urology & Continence Care Today*, up to 80 percent of postmenopausal women report some of a cluster of symptoms referred to as genitourinary syndrome of menopause (GSM).[5]
- **Mood changes**, including increased anxiety, irritability, or depressive symptoms. These emotional shifts are attributed to diminished amounts of estrogen, which plays an important role in influencing the neurotransmitters, such as serotonin and dopamine, that regulate mood.
- **Cognitive disturbances** such as memory lapses, reduced focus, or "brain fog." While these are usually temporary, studies show that they can interfere with daily functioning and productivity.
- **Musculoskeletal pain, joint stiffness, and changes in skin elasticity and hydration (dry skin)**, which are linked to collagen loss due to lower estrogen.

From a metabolic perspective, menopause often contributes to changes in body composition. Women may experience increased central fat deposition in the abdomen, bloating, and a decline in lean muscle mass. In fact, a 2022 study published in *Women's Health Reports* found that postmenopausal women had significantly greater visceral fat accumulation, even when controlling for age and overall body weight, and that this increases the risk for cardiovascular disease.[6]

Sleep disturbances also become more common during menopause due to the interplay of vasomotor symptoms (hot flashes and sweating), declining melatonin (the "sleep" hormone), and age-related changes in circadian rhythm. Up to 60 percent of menopausal women report difficulty falling or staying asleep, according to data from SWAN.[7]

Menopause is not just a short-lived, inconsequential phase but a pivotal period for assessing and preparing for long-term health. While many menopausal symptoms can be temporary and eventually resolve, they can be serious, as the sharp decline in estrogen can also cause long-term consequences that increase a woman's risk for chronic conditions including:

- **Osteoporosis:** Bone density loss accelerates during and immediately after menopause due to the dramatic drop in estrogen.
- **Cardiovascular disease:** Estrogen plays a protective role in vascular health, and thus its absence increases the risk of cardiovascular disease.
- **Type 2 diabetes and metabolic syndrome:** Hormonal changes, including a decline in estrogen levels, can impair insulin sensitivity.
- **Cognitive decline:** Estrogen is involved in nerve cell repair and function, and its loss may contribute to increased risk for Alzheimer's disease in genetically predisposed women.

Understanding the breadth of changes that occur during menopause allows for targeted strategies—both preventive and therapeutic—to enhance quality of life and safeguard long-term health. This period is often one of reflection and reset, providing the opportunity to prioritize health, reassess goals, and embrace a new phase of empowered living.

Menopause and Its Biological Impact

Biologically, menopause signals the end of ovarian follicular activity. With the cessation of ovulation comes a dramatic drop in estrogen and progesterone levels, causing noticeable physiological shifts.

- More frequent or intense hot flashes
- Vaginal dryness and decreased libido
- Joint and muscle pain
- Urinary tract symptoms and incontinence
- Mood disorders or emotional instability

POSTMENOPAUSE

Postmenopause is defined as the time after a woman has been without a period for twelve months. This phase lasts the rest of a woman's life. As life expectancy continues to rise, many women, depending on how long they live, will spend one-third to one-half of their lives in postmenopause, making it essential to understand the physiological, emotional, and preventive care needs that arise during this time.

Biologically, postmenopause is characterized by persistently low levels of estrogen and progesterone. While these hormones stabilize after fluctuating in perimenopause and dropping steeply during menopause, they eventually settle and remain far below reproductive levels. The body must adapt to this new hormonal baseline, and these adaptations influence nearly every organ system—from bones and the brain to the heart, skin, and urogenital tract.

Thankfully, for many women, most of the acute symptoms experienced during perimenopause and menopause—such as hot flashes, mood swings, and sleep disturbances—begin to dramatically diminish, becoming less frequent or totally disappearing. However, other symptoms—particularly those linked to long-term estrogen deficiency—may persist or emerge more prominently. These can include vaginal atrophy (vaginal walls become dry, thin, and inflamed), reduced bone density, weight gain, and a higher risk of chronic disease. While the experience varies greatly among individuals, this phase brings important health considerations that can benefit from proactive planning and supportive care.

Key physiological and clinical concerns that you should be aware of during this stage include:

- **Accelerated bone loss and osteoporosis risk:** Estrogen plays a crucial role in regulating bone remodeling. With its decline, bone resorption (breakdown of bone) exceeds bone formation, leading to increased risk of osteopenia (reduced bone mass of lesser severity than osteoporosis) and osteoporosis. According to the Bone Health and Osteoporosis Foundation, up to 50 percent of women over age fifty will experience an osteoporosis-related fracture in their lifetime.[8] Data also shows that women can lose up to 20 percent of their bone density in the five to seven years following menopause.
- **Higher incidence of cardiovascular disease:** Estrogen contributes to protection against cardiovascular disease by helping to keep

the arteries soft and flexible and promoting the healthy regulation of fats (lipids) by raising the levels of HDL ("good" cholesterol) and lowering levels of LDL ("bad" cholesterol). This is important, because it means postmenopausal women are at greater risk of developing hypertension, atherosclerosis (collection of fatty plaques along the inner walls of arteries), and coronary artery disease (disease of the blood vessels that feed the heart). A study in *Circulation* reported a marked increase in cardiovascular risk in women within the first ten years postmenopause.[9] A meta-analysis in *JAMA Cardiology* found that postmenopausal women have a 50 percent higher risk of developing heart disease compared to premenopausal women of the same age.[10]

- **Continued genitourinary symptoms (GSM):** Vaginal dryness, itching, pain during intercourse, and urinary urgency or incontinence may persist or worsen with the sharp decline in estrogen levels. These symptoms result from thinning of the vaginal and urethral tissues and decreased local blood flow. The pelvic floor muscles may also weaken, contributing to urgency and stress incontinence. Additionally, reduced lubrication and changes in pH increase the risk of urinary tract infections and discomfort during intercourse.
- **Changes in skin elasticity and hair thinning:** Estrogen supports collagen production, hydration, and skin thickness. Its absence contributes to fine lines, sagging skin, and increased sensitivity. Hair may also thin due to decreased follicular support and changes in the ratio of androgen to estrogen.
- **Cognitive changes and dementia risk:** Some women report increased forgetfulness or difficulty concentrating. Estrogen supports the health of the neurotransmitter system that includes serotonin,

dopamine, and acetylcholine, which are essential for mood, memory, and cognition. A drop in estrogen levels has been linked in brain imaging studies in postmenopausal women to a decrease in brain metabolism and shrinkage in an important area of the brain called the hippocampus, which is responsible for learning and memory. A 2023 study published in *eClinicalMedicine* suggested that women who undergo early menopause are at increased risk for dementia and deteriorating brain health.[11]

- **Weight gain and metabolic shifts:** Menopause often brings about a redistribution of body fat, particularly central adiposity (abdominal fat), due to a drop in estrogen and reduced basal metabolic rate. This visceral fat is associated with insulin resistance and increased inflammation. A study in the journal *Nutrients* underscores that postmenopausal women accumulate abdominal fat at a rate nearly twice that of premenopausal women under similar dietary conditions.[12]

Despite these challenges, postmenopause can also be a time of renewal and empowerment. Many women report experiencing a profound shift in priorities, self-confidence, and well-being. The freedom from menstrual cycles and reproductive anxiety opens the door for renewed energy, creativity, and sharpened focus on personal goals.

With proactive health strategies—including weight-bearing exercise, bone health monitoring, cardiovascular screening, pelvic floor therapy, and a nutrient-rich diet—postmenopausal women can optimize longevity and quality of life. Health literacy, regular checkups, and open dialogue with providers are essential to thriving in this dynamic phase.

Postmenopause is not a biological afterthought. It is an important and potentially transformative chapter in a woman's health journey.

Common Symptoms by Menopause Stage

Symptom	Perimenopause	Menopause	Postmenopause
Hot Flashes	✓	✓✓	✓
Mood Swings	✓	✓	
Sleep Issues	✓	✓✓	✓
Weight Gain	✓	✓✓	✓✓
Vaginal Dryness		✓	✓✓
Bone Loss		✓	✓✓

✓ Indicates that the symptom is present or occasionally experienced during that stage. It may be mild or intermittent.

✓✓ Indicates that the symptom is more common, frequent, or severe during that stage. It typically affects a larger proportion of women and/or presents with greater intensity.

A CLOSER LOOK AT ESTROGEN AND PROGESTERONE'S ROLE IN MENOPAUSE-RELATED CONDITIONS

Menopause is primarily driven by the gradual loss of ovarian follicles and the resultant decrease in estrogen and progesterone. As discussed earlier, these hormones don't just influence the menstrual cycle. They impact nearly every part of the body, including the brain, heart, bones, skin, and urogenital system. Understanding menopause means recognizing the consequences of hormonal decline as it relates particularly to these hormones.

Estrogen and progesterone are the two primary sex hormones in the female body. Both are steroid hormones, meaning they are derived from cholesterol and have the power to influence countless physiological systems. Estrogen is often associated with traditionally feminine characteristics such as breast development and fat distribution, while progesterone is more directly involved in preparing the body for pregnancy and helping to stabilize the effects of estrogen.

These hormones are predominantly produced in the ovaries. Estrogen is synthesized by the ovarian follicles in the first half of the menstrual cycle, though it is also constantly being made in smaller amounts by the adrenal glands and, after menopause, by fat tissue. During pregnancy, the placenta becomes a major source of estrogen. Progesterone, on the other hand, is produced primarily by the corpus luteum—a temporary structure that forms in the ovary after ovulation. Like estrogen, progesterone is also produced in the adrenal glands, and during pregnancy, it's made in significant quantities by the placenta.

Estrogen performs a wide variety of roles in the body, as mentioned earlier. It is a multifunctional hormone that affects nearly every organ system in the body. It regulates the menstrual cycle by stimulating the thickening of the uterine lining and plays a crucial role in the development of secondary sex characteristics during puberty. It also contributes to the maintenance of bone density and enhances skin elasticity. Additionally, estrogen influences brain function and mood regulation by modulating neurotransmitters such as serotonin, dopamine, and acetylcholine, which are essential for mood stability, memory, and emotional regulation. In the cardiovascular system, estrogen promotes vasodilation, reduces arterial stiffness, and helps maintain a favorable lipid profile by increasing HDL and decreasing LDL.

In the central nervous system, estrogen has neuroprotective effects, enhancing cerebral blood flow, reducing inflammation, and stimulating the growth of neurons and synapses. Studies suggest that estrogen may protect against neurodegenerative diseases, although the timing and type of estrogen exposure are critical in determining its benefits.

Progesterone's primary role is to prepare the uterus for the potential implantation of a fertilized egg and to maintain a pregnancy in its early stages. It plays a vital role in modulating the actions of estrogen to prevent excessive tissue growth. Beyond reproductive health, it acts as a natural calming hormone in the brain: supporting mood stability, reducing anxiety, and promoting restorative sleep by enhancing the effects of the neurotransmitter GABA (gamma-aminobutyric acid). Progesterone also helps counterbalance estrogen's stimulatory effects, contributing to hormonal harmony and reducing symptoms such as breast tenderness, bloating, and headaches when estrogen is high. In addition, it supports bone health by working alongside estrogen to regulate bone turnover, helping maintain bone density over time. Progesterone influences metabolic health as well, aiding in blood sugar regulation and supporting thyroid hormone action at the cellular level. Its anti-inflammatory and diuretic properties further assist with fluid balance and immune modulation, making progesterone an essential hormone for neurological health, metabolic stability, and overall well-being throughout a woman's lifespan, not just during the reproductive years.

These two hormones work together in a coordinated cycle. During the follicular phase of the menstrual cycle (the first fourteen days), estrogen levels rise, promoting the growth of the uterine lining. Around day fourteen, this rise triggers ovulation. After ovulation, during the luteal phase, progesterone levels increase to stabilize and prepare the lining for a possible pregnancy. If pregnancy does not occur, both hormone levels drop, leading to menstruation. Estrogen and progesterone work in a harmonious relationship—estrogen stimulates and builds, while progesterone calms and balances.

However, during menopause, the hormonal balance between estrogen and progesterone shifts dramatically. The ovaries gradually reduce hormone production, particularly after ovulation ceases. Progesterone is often the first hormone to decline significantly, due to the lack of corpus luteum formation. Estrogen, especially estradiol—the most potent form of estrogen—also drops substantially. This hormonal decline contributes to many of the hallmark symptoms of menopause, including hot flashes, night sweats, mood swings, vaginal dryness, and sleep disturbances, and to greater long-term risk of osteoporosis and cardiovascular disease. As hormone levels stabilize at new, lower levels during postmenopause, the body enters a new phase of hormonal regulation with far-reaching physiological implications.

Understanding the origin, function, and interaction of estrogen and progesterone provides a foundational perspective for navigating not just the changes that occur during menopause, but also the interventions that might be considered to counterbalance them. These interventions will take different forms and can be combined for maximal benefit. Some are nutritional, others are physical, and the rest are lifestyle behavior modifications.

Functions of Estrogen and Progesterone in the Body

System	Estrogen	Progesterone
Reproductive System	• Stimulates growth of uterine lining (endometrium) • Promotes development of secondary sex characteristics • Regulates menstrual cycle	• Prepares endometrium for implantation • Maintains pregnancy • Prevents uterine contractions during early pregnancy • Regulates menstrual cycle by opposing estrogen's proliferative effects
Skeletal System	• Supports bone formation and density • Reduces bone resorption	• Supports bone metabolism (less direct role than estrogen)
Cardiovascular System	• Promotes vasodilation • Maintains healthy cholesterol levels	• Has a mild vasodilatory effect • Supports blood vessel integrity

System	Estrogen	Progesterone
Nervous System	• Enhances mood and cognitive function • Modulates serotonin and dopamine	• Has calming, anti-anxiety effects • Modulates GABA receptors
Skin and Hair	• Maintains skin thickness and elasticity • Promotes hair growth	• Supports skin hydration and barrier repair
Metabolism	• Improves insulin sensitivity • Influences fat distribution (stored in hips/thighs)	• Increases basal body temperature • Supports metabolic rate in luteal phase
Immune System	• Modulates immune responses • Has anti-inflammatory effects	• Promotes immune tolerance in pregnancy • Supports mucosal immunity
Urinary Tract	• Maintains bladder and urethral tissue integrity	• Supports urogenital tissue maintenance
Breast Tissue	• Stimulates breast development during puberty and pregnancy	• Prepares breasts for milk production • Opposes excessive growth

WHY MENOPAUSE-RELATED CONDITIONS OCCUR

When hormone levels fall, the systems they once regulated must find a new equilibrium, because estrogen plays a crucial role in numerous physiological functions, and its withdrawal during menopause contributes to a complex cascade of systemic changes, affecting everything from bone metabolism to fat distribution and blood vessel elasticity. This hormonal vacuum impacts multiple organ systems in ways that were discussed earlier: increased osteoporosis risk, increased risk for cardiovascular disease, urinary incontinence/urogenital atrophy, cognitive and neurological shifts, weight gain, and metabolic changes. Understanding why these symptoms occur is critical in understanding how treatments and other interventions are designed to help manage or mitigate them.

MANAGING MENOPAUSE: AN OVERVIEW OF VARIOUS APPROACHES

The good news is that while menopause is inevitable, suffering is not. A comprehensive and integrative approach allows women to address symptoms and enhance long-term wellness. Although this book's focus is on the role nutrition can play in the management of menopause, understanding the full range of available options empowers women to choose strategies aligned with their unique medical profiles, cultural preferences, and lifestyle goals. These approaches can be categorized into four primary modalities: hormone replacement therapy, nonhormonal medications, complementary and alternative medicine (CAM), and lifestyle interventions. Women are best advised to understand these options as best as possible, then talk to their private healthcare provider about which, if any, are suitable for them.

Hormone Replacement Therapy (HRT)

HRT involves the administration of estrogen—either alone (for women without a uterus) or combined with progesterone (for women with a uterus)—to supplement the body's declining hormone levels. It remains the most effective treatment for relieving hot flashes, night sweats, and vaginal dryness and preventing bone loss. Beyond symptom relief, HRT may provide cardioprotective and neuroprotective benefits when started near the onset of menopause. Forms of HRT include pills, patches, gels, vaginal rings, and creams. The choice depends on a woman's symptoms, health profile, and preferences. Transdermal (patch) estrogen may carry fewer risks than oral forms and is preferred for women with higher risks for abnormal blood clotting.

Large studies like the Women's Health Initiative (WHI) once raised concerns about breast cancer and cardiovascular risks, but current evaluations suggest that for healthy women under age sixty or within ten years of menopause, the benefits of HRT outweigh the risks. Individualized risk assessment is critical and should consider personal and family history of breast cancer, stroke, and thromboembolic (traveling blood clots) events. These are all things to be discussed with your doctor or other healthcare provider.

Nonhormonal Medications

For women who cannot or choose not to use HRT, several nonhormonal pharmaceutical options are available. These can address vasomotor symptoms, mood disturbances, and sleep issues without affecting estrogen levels.

- **SSRIs (Selective Serotonin Reuptake Inhibitors) and SNRIs (Serotonin Norepinephrine Reuptake Inhibitors):** Medications such as paroxetine, venlafaxine, and escitalopram, which treat depression and anxiety disorders, have been shown to reduce the frequency and severity of hot flashes by 50–60 percent. They also can improve mood disorders that are common in perimenopausal women.
- **Gabapentin:** Originally an anti-seizure drug, gabapentin has been shown in randomized clinical trials to be especially helpful in women who experience night sweats and hot flashes.

- **Clonidine:** This is an older antihypertensive medication that can modestly reduce vasomotor symptoms, although it can also result in side effects like dry mouth and dizziness.
- **Ospemifene:** This selective estrogen receptor modulator (SERM) is approved for the treatment of painful intercourse due to vaginal atrophy and offers a non-estrogen alternative to treat urogenital symptoms.

Like any medication, each of these alternatives should be considered in consultation with a healthcare provider to weigh efficacy, side effects, and interactions with other medications.

Complementary and Alternative Medicine (CAM)

Many women turn to natural and integrative approaches for managing menopausal symptoms. While scientific support of these different treatments varies, some therapies have demonstrated promise in clinical trials. There has not been universally consistent data that shows these therapies have worked for all or even most women, but there has been a tremendous amount of self-reporting indicating that many women have found some benefit. Take this information in concert with advice from your healthcare provider and decide if any of these strategies might be right for you.

- **Phytoestrogens:** Found in soy, flaxseed, red clover, and legumes, phytoestrogens mimic the structure of estrogen and can weakly bind to estrogen receptors. Meta-analyses suggest their consumption can lead to modest reductions in hot flash frequency and intensity, particularly with consistent use over twelve or more weeks.
- **Black cohosh:** Black cohosh is a North American perennial herb that has long been used in traditional medicine for gynecological issues and to support women's reproductive health, especially by

Indigenous peoples and later in Western herbalism. Some studies show it can help reduce hot flashes, though results are mixed, and it may not be effective long term.

- **Acupuncture:** Acupuncture is a key component of traditional Chinese medicine that involves the insertion of fine needles into specific points on the body to stimulate energy flow, or "qi." It is based on the belief that balancing this flow of energy promotes health and alleviates disease. Randomized controlled trials suggest that acupuncture may help regulate vasomotor symptoms, anxiety, and sleep, though it's still unclear how effective it really is for menopausal women.
- **Mindfulness-based stress reduction (MBSR):** Programs like yoga, meditation, and tai chi reduce cortisol levels, improve sleep, and support emotional regulation. While cortisol is an important hormone that counteracts stress, and has many functionalities including increasing blood sugar levels, reducing inflammation, increasing blood pressure, and stimulating the immune system, too much cortisol can cause problems, such as increasing inflammation, weight gain, fatigue, insomnia, high blood pressure, high blood sugar, and thinning skin. A notable randomized control trial showed that MBSR may be a clinically significant resource in reducing the degree of bother and distress women experience from hot flashes and night sweats.[13]
- **Evening primrose oil and dong quai:** These herbal supplements are popular but have less robust clinical support. Dong quai is a traditional Chinese medicinal herb often referred to as the "female ginseng" due to its historical use in treating women's health issues—especially those related to hormonal balance. Evening primrose oil is extracted from the seeds of the *Oenothera biennis* plant and has been heralded by some for its potential anti-inflammatory properties, though strong scientific evidence is limited. Use of these

therapies should be discussed with a provider, especially if you're taking anticoagulants or hormone-sensitive medications.

CAM therapies are best used as part of an integrative plan and monitored for safety and interactions.

Lifestyle Interventions

Lifestyle changes are foundational to managing menopausal symptoms and enhancing long-term health. They offer holistic benefits that extend beyond symptom relief and help reduce the risk of chronic disease. The following are some behavioral choices that many women have made and found to be beneficial.

- **Nutrition:** A Mediterranean or anti-inflammatory diet rich in leafy greens, berries, whole grains, legumes, and omega-3 fatty acids supports hormonal balance and reduces inflammation. Nutrient priorities include calcium (1,200 mg/day), vitamin D (600–800 IU), magnesium, and fiber. Understanding how these and other nutrients play a role in your management of menopausal symptoms is the cornerstone of this book. There are some variables that will be out of your control, but nutrient intake is something you can customize and own.
- **Exercise:** Engaging in regular physical activity—especially resistance training, walking, yoga, and Pilates—improves mood, reduces hot flashes, maintains bone density, and supports cardiovascular health. Vast research has demonstrated the benefits of at least 150 minutes of moderate-intensity aerobic activity per week, along with 2–3 sessions of strength training. In fact, the Women's Health Initiative study showed that physically active women had a lower risk of hip fractures and total fractures overall.[14] While

nutrition is the core of this book, exercise plays a significant role and gets its time in the spotlight in the coming chapters.

- **Weight management:** Maintaining a healthy weight can reduce vasomotor symptoms and improve metabolic health. Avoiding excess alcohol, sugar, and refined carbohydrates can stabilize blood glucose and energy.
- **Sleep hygiene:** Sleep disturbances affect up to 60 percent of menopausal women. Establishing a consistent bedtime, limiting caffeine and screen exposure, and practicing relaxation techniques can improve sleep quality.
- **Stress reduction:** Chronic stress amplifies cortisol and exacerbates menopause symptoms. Techniques like deep breathing, gratitude journaling, and spending time in nature can buffer these effects.
- **Social connection:** Support networks—whether through peer groups, therapy, or online forums—have been shown to improve emotional resilience and overall satisfaction during this life transition.

Making even small changes in these areas can significantly improve quality of life and reduce long-term health risks.

THE ROLE OF MEDICATIONS, SUPPLEMENTS, AND NUTRITION

There is no single approach to addressing the symptoms and challenges of the menopausal period. Because every woman experiences menopause differently, the strategies that will work can be different for different individuals. Using medications and supplements is a personal choice that should be made in consultation with your healthcare provider. There are lots of pros and cons, and thoughtful discussions can help you make decisions that are best and most comfortable for you.

Nutritional changes, however, can be adopted by anyone. They are not just the foundation for a better menopause, but the bedrock of your overall health and quality of life. They're also something you can directly choose and control, which gives you greater agency in alleviating your symptoms and improving various biochemical markers that reflect the occurrence or risk for disease.

Some women might choose a multifaceted approach to symptom relief by combining two or more of the general strategies. Many women take medications and supplements, while others just take one or the other. Regardless of which combination you choose, adding nutritional changes to these can be helpful in bringing you the relief and comfort that you seek.

The nutrients that are emphasized later in the book are nature's remedies and helpers for many of the challenges faced before, during, and after menopause, particularly those brought on by the hormonal shifts. Some women might even choose to deal with the challenges of menopause entirely through the foods they eat and a regular exercise program. It's important that you choose what fits your lifestyle and works best for you.

REDEFINING THE NARRATIVE AROUND MENOPAUSE

Culturally, menopause has often been viewed through a lens of loss—loss of youth, fertility, and vibrancy. But this chapter in a woman's life can also be a time of incredible growth, self-discovery, and empowerment. Menopause is a portal to a new era in life, a time when many women reevaluate priorities, embrace self-care, and step into their power.

Rather than viewing menopause as an end, it's time to reframe it as a profound transformation—biologically, emotionally, and socially. Many women find that once the fog of hormonal chaos clears, they are left with a stronger sense of self and a desire to prioritize their well-being. Midlife offers a renewed opportunity for self-reflection, realignment, and growth.

Studies show that psychological well-being often improves postmenopause, particularly among women who have access to education, community support, and healthcare.[15] This chapter in life can be rich with vitality. Women in their fifties, sixties, and beyond are increasingly becoming leaders, mentors, innovators, and cultural influencers, and the narrative must evolve to match that reality.

Reframing menopause doesn't mean dismissing its challenges, rather it means recognizing the strength, resilience, and wisdom that emerge through navigating them. Empowerment comes from education. The more we understand what happens to the body and why, the better prepared we are to make informed, personalized decisions. By understanding the science, knowing what to expect, and taking proactive steps—nutritionally, physically, and emotionally—women can approach menopause with clarity and confidence. Menopause is not a medical failure to be endured but a natural evolution to be embraced.

The rest of this book will explore in greater depth the most effective nutritional, behavioral, and environmental strategies for optimizing health through this transition. But for now, remember this: Menopause is not the proverbial end, rather it's the transition to a new beginning—a biological reset that with the right knowledge and tools can launch a healthier, wiser, more empowered chapter of life.

2

MIDLIFE POWER NUTRIENTS

At midlife, your body begins writing a new chapter—one in which the rules of health, metabolism, and energy undergo significant revision. The hormonal symphony that once played in harmony—sustaining fertility, bone strength, heart health, and cognitive clarity—starts to quiet, shift, and sometimes stutter. Estrogen, the powerful modulator of dozens of physiological systems, begins its gradual decline, and with it, the body enters a vulnerable yet powerful phase of transformation. With the right tools, this becomes an opportunity for a reset, and one of the most powerful tools we have is food.

The nutrients you consume in midlife matter more than ever, because nutrients are not just fuel. They actively participate in your biology. They instruct your cells, protect your DNA, rebalance your hormones, and modulate the inflammation and oxidative stress (harmful effects caused by the accumulation of reactive oxygen species in the body) that accelerate the aging process. Every bite of food you take contains molecular information that can either support the body's natural resilience to disease or contribute to the breakdown of one or more of the body's complex systems.

Menopause can bring with it an array of challenges: fatigue, mood swings, hot flashes, joint pain, brain fog, sleep disruption, and increased risk for chronic diseases like osteoporosis, cardiovascular disease, type 2 diabetes, and cognitive decline. What unites these challenges is that they all represent disrupted physiology—something the right nutrients can influence and, in many instances, reverse with precision and care.

Unlike most medications, nutrients work synergistically and gradually. They support the body's built-in healing processes and provide the basics for rebuilding neurotransmitters restoring hormone sensitivity, repairing tissue, and fueling your mitochondria—the tiny energy factories inside your cells. In other words, nutrients do not mask symptoms, rather they address their source.

Additionally, our nutrient needs increase in midlife, even as the number of calories we need tends to decrease. This means the food we eat must be more concentrated in nutrients and smarter in function. This is especially true in the face of common midlife nutritional challenges such as lower digestive enzyme output, reduced stomach acid, declining vitamin D synthesis from sun exposure, and shifting taste and appetite signals.

Nutrition also becomes a cornerstone of mental resilience. Several nutrients play key roles in mood regulation, memory, and sleep, areas that are often disturbed during perimenopause and beyond. For example, magnesium calms the nervous system, B vitamins energize the brain, and omega-3 fatty acids reduce anxiety and support memory consolidation. These aren't trivial benefits, as they are essential for maintaining a sense of self, productivity, and calm. Yet, most women are never told that what they eat can profoundly shape their menopausal experience. They are offered prescriptions, given over-the-counter hormone creams, or simply told, "This is just part of getting older." But by adding a nutrient-based approach to their daily regimen, many women have learned that they can relieve symptoms, prevent long-term disease, and revitalize their body without relying solely on pharmaceutical intervention.

During perimenopause, menopause, and postmenopause, women must pay attention to not only the types of nutrients they are consuming but also the quantity. There are certain nutrients women need to consume in greater quantities than they did earlier in life. Younger women have more flexibility and better ability to recover when they do not get enough nutrients, but as we age, nutrient deficiencies can have a more damaging impact on our health in a shorter period of time.

Vitamin D requirements provide a good example of how recommendations change during this stage of life. They increase with age for several reasons, including the higher risk of osteoporosis, increased cardiovascular disease risk, and decreased estrogen level, which impairs the body's ability to absorb calcium and produce vitamin D on its own.

Life Stage	Vitamin D Recommended Daily Amount
Premenopause	600 IU
Perimenopause	600 IU
Menopause	600 IU
Postmenopause	800 IU

Source: Endocrine Society

Calcium is another important nutrient whose recommendations change depending on the life stage.

Life Stage	Calcium Recommended Daily Amount
Premenopause and Perimenopause	1,000 mg/day
Menopause and Postmenopause	1,200 mg/day

Note that these values as well as other recommendations throughout the book might differ based on an individual's specific health conditions and other factors, so consult your healthcare provider for your specific recommendations.

There are many nutrients that women should consider increasing during these stages of life. While the following lists are not comprehensive, they cover the most important nutrients and are a good start when considering the changes that need to be made. Note that just because a nutrient is not listed for a particular stage, it doesn't mean that nutrient is not beneficial in that stage. The lists are meant to emphasize what stands out as most relevant for that stage. For example, antioxidants are important during ALL phases and ages of life, but they might be a bigger priority at different times for different reasons. Thus, just because it's not listed doesn't mean it isn't still important and beneficial.

Perimenopause and Menopause

Nutrient	Why It Matters	Some Key Sources
B Vitamins (B6, B9, B12)	Support energy, cognition, and cardiovascular health	Eggs, fortified cereals, leafy greens
Calcium	Counteracts bone loss due to declining estrogen levels	Dairy, fortified drinks, greens, tofu
Magnesium	Works with vitamin D and calcium for improved bone and muscle health	Beans, greens (e.g., spinach), legumes, seeds (e.g., pumpkin seeds)
Omega-3 Fatty Acids (EPA/DHA)	Improve lipid profile, reduce hot flashes	Algae oil, flaxseed, salmon, sardines
Phytoestrogens (Isoflavones, Lignans)	Gently mimic estrogen, ease hot flashes	Chickpeas, flaxseed, soy
Protein	Prevents muscle loss (sarcopenia), stabilizes blood sugar	Beans, eggs, fish, lentils, tofu, yogurt
Vitamin D	Essential for calcium absorption and bone remodeling	Fatty fish (e.g., salmon), fortified foods, sunlight, supplements
Vitamin K2	Directs calcium into bones instead of arteries	Eggs, fermented soy (natto), hard cheese

Postmenopause

Nutrient	Why It Matters	Some Key Sources
Antioxidants (C, E, Zinc, Selenium)	Protect cells, skin, and immune function	Berries, citrus, nuts, whole grains
Calcium	Maintains bone mass and prevents osteoporosis	Dairy, fortified drinks, greens, tofu
Choline	Supports memory, cognition, and liver health	Eggs, salmon, soybeans
Fiber	Lowers cholesterol, supports gut health and weight loss	Legumes, oats, vegetables
Magnesium	Aids bone formation, sleep, and blood pressure	Beans, greens (e.g., spinach), legumes, seeds (e.g., pumpkin seeds)
Omega-3 Fatty Acids (EPA/DHA)	Protect heart, brain, and joints	Algae oil, flaxseed, salmon, sardines
Protein	Preserves lean mass, prevents metabolic slowdown	Beans, eggs, fish, lentils, tofu, yogurt
Vitamin D	Enhances calcium absorption, supports immunity	Fatty fish (e.g., salmon), fortified foods, sunlight, supplements
Vitamin K2	Directs calcium to bones, prevents arterial calcification	Eggs, fermented soy (natto), hard cheese

THE WISDOM ISN'T NEW, IT'S ANCIENT

Traditional cultures have long known that food is medicine, and that its healing capacity intensifies during major life transitions like menopause. In traditional Chinese medicine, menopause has long been treated as a deficiency of yin and blood—conditions nourished by mineral-rich broths, black sesame seeds, soy products, and warming spices like ginger and cinnamon. Ayurvedic medicine, practiced for over three thousand years in India, views menopause as a natural shift in the doshas (the three fundamental energies that govern our body, mind, and behavior), and dietary therapies include ghee (a purified butter rich in fat-soluble vitamins), dates, sesame, and adaptogenic herbs to stabilize mood and energy. Even ancient Greek medicine, pioneered by Hippocrates—the father of Western medicine—emphasized that food should be our "first medicine," and used plant-based preparations rich in phytoestrogens, iron, and calcium from herbs, legumes, and leafy greens to treat women's hormonal imbalances.

These practices weren't mystical, rather they were observational sciences grounded in pattern recognition. Now, centuries later, those patterns are confirmed by controlled studies, biochemical analysis, and medical imaging.

YOUR BODY IS CHANGING—YOUR NUTRITIONAL STRATEGY SHOULD, TOO

During the reproductive years, your body operated under a specific hormonal template. Estrogen did more than regulate your cycle; it protected your heart, brain, bones, skin, and metabolism. When estrogen declines, your nutrient needs change accordingly. While you may no longer need as many calories, your nutritional needs increase sharply. That means every meal must now work harder for you. Food must not just fill you up—it must replenish, rebuild, and reprogram. Do not mistake this as being a time about restriction or deprivation. In fact, it's quite the opposite. It's about liberation—freeing yourself from the roller coaster of symptoms and reclaiming your energy, clarity, and strength through smarter nourishment.

This chapter will introduce the most scientifically supported nutrients for menopausal women and explain how each can help regulate specific symptoms, protect long-term health, and restore biological balance. For each nutrient, we'll identify: (1) why it matters during menopause, (2) what symptoms it supports or prevents, (3) how much is typically needed to see results, and (4) which foods provide the richest, most accessible sources.

You'll also find a comprehensive table of foods to limit or avoid—not because we're chasing perfection, but because certain ingredients work against the body's efforts to adapt during this transition. Think of this chapter as both a guide and a toolbox. You don't have to memorize everything, but by the end, you'll understand which nutrients to prioritize and how to build meals that are functional, flavorful, and fiercely supportive of your future health. Remember that food, when chosen wisely and eaten consistently, becomes more than sustenance—it becomes medicine, protection, and power.

Nutrients for Symptom Relief

Symptom	Helpful Nutrient
Bone Loss	Calcium, Magnesium, Vitamin B2, Vitamin D
Brain Fog and Memory Lapses	Folate, Omega-3s, Vitamin B12
Fatigue	Iron, Magnesium, Vitamin B Complex
Hot Flashes	Omega-3s, Phytoestrogens, Vitamin E
Insomnia	Calcium, Magnesium, Vitamin D
Joint Pain	Magnesium, Omega-3s, Vitamin D
Mood Swings and Irritability	Magnesium, Omega-3s, Vitamin B Complex
Vaginal Dryness	Omega-3s, Vitamin E, Zinc

CALCIUM: THE BONE KEEPER

Why It Matters

Calcium is the most abundant mineral in the human body, with over 99 percent stored in the bones and teeth. As estrogen levels drop during menopause, the rate of bone resorption (breakdown) begins to exceed the rate of bone formation, and this leads to decreased bone density and a heightened risk of osteoporosis and fractures. Estrogen acts as a key regulator of bone turnover by suppressing the activity of osteoclasts, which are the cells responsible for breaking down bone tissue. When estrogen declines, osteoclast activity increases, causing bones to lose density more rapidly. Adequate calcium intake becomes essential to offset this loss and maintain bone integrity.

While calcium might be most famous for its role in bone health, its activities extend well beyond our skeleton. It also has a crucial function in muscle contractions (including the heart), nerve transmission, blood clotting, and hormonal secretion. Without sufficient calcium, menopausal women may experience muscle cramps, brittle nails, dental decay, and even abnormal heart rhythms. It's also worth noting that, in general, as vitamin D levels fall (often due to less sun exposure), calcium absorption from the food we eat is impaired, making both nutrients jointly essential (see next section).

Symptom Relief and Prevention

- Supports nerve conduction and muscle function
- Aids blood clotting and cardiac rhythm
- Prevents osteoporosis

Recommended Intake

1,200 mg/day for women over fifty

Notable Food Sources of Calcium

Food	Calcium Content
Almonds	76 mg per oz
Amaranth (cooked)	116 mg per cup
Blackstrap molasses	172 mg per tbsp
Broccoli (cooked)	62 mg per cup
Cheddar cheese	200 mg per oz
Chia seeds	179 mg per oz
Collard greens (cooked)	268 mg per cup
Figs (dried)	121 mg per ½ cup
Fortified almond milk	450 mg per cup

Food	Calcium Content
Fortified orange juice	300 mg per cup
Kale (cooked)	94 mg per cup
Mustard greens (cooked)	165 mg per cup
Navy beans	126 mg per cup
Okra (cooked)	82 mg per cup
Quinoa (cooked)	31 mg per cup
Rhubarb (cooked)	105 mg per cup
Sardines (with bones)	325 mg per 3 oz
Sesame seeds	88 mg per tbsp
Soybeans (cooked)	175 mg per cup
Tempeh	184 mg per cup
Tofu (calcium-set)	253 mg per ½ cup
Turnip greens (cooked)	197 mg per cup
Wakame seaweed	150 mg per ½ cup
White beans (cooked)	161 mg per cup
Yogurt (plain, low-fat)	415 mg per cup

VITAMIN D: THE SUNSHINE ALLY

Why It Matters

Vitamin D is a fat-soluble vitamin (meaning it dissolves and gets stored in fat) that functions more like a hormone than a traditional nutrient. It's produced in the skin in response to UVB rays from sunlight, and it's vital for regulating calcium and phosphate metabolism in the body. During menopause, when bone density is already compromised due to lower estrogen levels, vitamin D can help ensure that dietary calcium is effectively absorbed from the gut. Without adequate vitamin D, even high-calcium diets can fail to protect bone integrity. The combination of calcium and vitamin D can provide a protective effect.

Beyond its role in calcium metabolism, vitamin D influences immune health, modulates inflammatory responses, and affects the nervous system. Low levels of vitamin D have been associated with increased risk of depression, cognitive decline, heart disease, and even autoimmune conditions—all of which become more prevalent with age and hormonal shifts. As estrogen has a neuroprotective and mood-regulating effect, its decline can leave women more vulnerable to mood disturbances and mental fog—both of which vitamin D may help buffer. Unfortunately, vitamin D deficiency is common in women over fifty, especially in those with limited sun exposure, darker skin tones, or gastrointestinal conditions that impair fat absorption.

Symptom Relief and Prevention

- Supports immune function
- Reduces depressive symptoms
- Prevents bone loss and fractures

Recommended Intake

600–800 IU/day (or higher if vitamin D deficient; consult your doctor)

Notable Food Sources of Vitamin D

Food	Vitamin D Content
Beef liver	49 IU per 3 oz
Butter	9 IU per tbsp
Caviar (black/red)	33 IU per tbsp
Cheese (Swiss)	12 IU per oz
Cod-liver oil	1,360 IU per tsp
Egg yolk	41 IU per large egg

Food	Vitamin D Content
Fortified almond milk	100 IU per cup
Fortified cereal	80–100 IU per serving
Fortified margarine	60 IU per tbsp
Fortified milk	120 IU per cup
Fortified orange juice	137 IU per cup
Fortified soy milk	100 IU per cup
Fortified tofu	80 IU per 3 oz
Halibut	190 IU per 3 oz
Herring (pickled)	680 IU per 3 oz
Mackerel	360 IU per 3 oz
Milk powder	100 IU per ¼ cup
Mushrooms (UV-exposed)	400 IU per ½ cup
Oysters	320 IU per 6 oysters
Ricotta cheese	25 IU per ½ cup
Salmon (sockeye)	570 IU per 3 oz
Sardines	270 IU per 3 oz
Shrimp	152 IU per 3 oz
Sole (baked)	104 IU per fillet
Tuna (canned in oil)	229 IU per 3 oz

MAGNESIUM:
THE MOOD AND MUSCLE MINERAL

Why It Matters

Magnesium is an essential mineral that serves as a cofactor in over three hundred enzymatic reactions in the body. It plays a critical role in nerve transmission, muscle contraction, glucose control, blood pressure regulation, and the synthesis of DNA, RNA, and proteins. During menopause, magnesium becomes particularly important due to its calming effect on the nervous system and its influence on hormone regulation.

Low magnesium levels have been linked to increased anxiety, irritability, sleep disturbances, and migraines, symptoms that often intensify during perimenopause and menopause. This mineral supports GABA (gamma-aminobutyric acid), the brain's primary inhibitory neurotransmitter, which helps quiet overactive neurons and promote relaxation. That's why magnesium is often referred to as nature's tranquilizer.

Additionally, magnesium is essential for maintaining cardiovascular health, which is a major concern postmenopause as estrogen's protective effects wane. It also helps regulate heart rhythm and blood pressure, and it's been shown to reduce systemic inflammation. Magnesium influences insulin sensitivity, making it crucial for managing the weight gain and metabolic changes that are common during midlife.

Symptom Relief and Prevention

- Improves sleep and reduces insomnia
- Eases anxiety and irritability
- Supports heart and bone health
- Helps with muscle cramps and headaches

Recommended Intake

320 mg/day

Notable Food Sources of Magnesium

Food	Magnesium Content
Almonds	77 mg per oz
Avocado	58 mg per fruit
Bananas	32 mg per medium
Barley (cooked)	35 mg per cup
Black beans (cooked)	120 mg per cup
Brazil nuts	107 mg per oz
Brown rice	84 mg per cup
Cashews	74 mg per oz
Chia seeds	95 mg per oz
Dark chocolate (70%–85%)	64 mg per oz
Edamame	99 mg per cup
Figs (dried)	25 mg per 2 pieces
Kale (cooked)	31 mg per cup
Lentils	71 mg per cup
Milk	24 mg per cup
Oatmeal	57 mg per cup
Peanuts	50 mg per oz
Potatoes (with skin)	43 mg per medium
Pumpkin seeds	168 mg per oz
Quinoa	118 mg per cup
Spinach (cooked)	157 mg per cup
Sunflower seeds	91 mg per oz
Swiss chard	150 mg per cup
Tofu	53 mg per ½ cup
Yogurt (plain, low-fat)	42 mg per cup

OMEGA-3 FATTY ACIDS: THE INFLAMMATION FIGHTERS

Why They Matter

Omega-3 fatty acids are polyunsaturated fats that play a critical role in reducing inflammation, maintaining brain function, and supporting cardiovascular health—particularly EPA (eicosapentaenoic acid) and DHA (docosahexaenoic acid). During menopause, the body enters a pro-inflammatory state due to decreased estrogen, which can exacerbate symptoms like joint pain, mood swings, and skin dryness. Omega-3s help counteract this shift by reducing inflammation.

Alpha-linoleic acid (ALA) is another essential omega-3 fatty acid. This plant-based antioxidant can only be obtained through the diet. It's associated with reduced risk for cardiovascular disease, less inflammation, and lower risk for Alzheimer's disease, dementia, and other cognitive issues.

These fatty acids also benefit cognitive function and mental well-being. DHA, in particular, is a major structural component of the brain. Several studies have shown that omega-3 intake correlates with reduced risk of depression, anxiety, and cognitive decline—conditions that many women find worsen with hormonal changes.

Cardiovascular risk increases postmenopause due to lipid profile changes (e.g., increases in LDL and triglycerides), and omega-3s help manage these markers by lowering triglyceride levels, reducing blood pressure, and improving the function of the cells lining the blood vessel walls. Their role in skin hydration and elasticity also makes them beneficial for combating the dry skin and loss of skin tone that can occur with estrogen depletion.

Symptom Relief and Prevention

- Reduce hot flashes (up to 55 percent, some studies suggest)
- Support cognitive function
- Protect heart health
- Help reduce joint stiffness and dry skin

Recommended Intake

ALA: 1.1–1.6 g/day
EPA/DHA: 250–500 mg/day

Notable Food Sources of Omega-3 Fatty Acids

Food	Omega-3 Content
Algae oil (supplement)	400–500 mg EPA/DHA
Anchovies	951 mg EPA/DHA per 3 oz
Beef (grass-fed)	80 mg EPA/DHA per 3 oz
Brussels sprouts	135 mg ALA per cup
Canola oil	1,300 mg ALA per tbsp
Caviar	1,080 mg EPA/DHA per tbsp
Chia seeds	5,060 mg ALA per oz
Edamame	280 mg ALA per ½ cup
Eggs (omega-3 enriched)	500 mg per large
Flaxseeds (ground)	6,400 mg ALA per 2 tbsp
Hemp seeds	6,000 mg ALA per 3 tbsp
Herring	3,100 mg EPA/DHA per 3 oz
Krill oil (supplement)	300–500 mg EPA/DHA
Mackerel	4,580 mg EPA/DHA per 3 oz
Natto	350 mg ALA per ½ cup

Food	Omega-3 Content
Oysters	720 mg EPA/DHA per 3 oz
Perilla oil	9,000 mg ALA per tbsp
Salmon (wild)	2,260 mg EPA/DHA per 3 oz
Sardines	2,200 mg EPA/DHA per 3 oz
Seaweed	Variable amounts
Soybeans	670 mg ALA per ½ cup
Spinach (raw)	41 mg ALA per cup
Tuna (bluefin)	2,100 mg EPA/DHA per 3 oz
Walnuts	2,570 mg ALA per oz
Winter squash	338 mg ALA per cup

B VITAMINS (B6, B9, B12): THE ENERGY REGULATORS

Why They Matter

The B vitamin family (B1, B2, B3, B5, B6, B7, B9, and B12) plays a central role in cellular energy production, red blood cell formation, brain function, and DNA synthesis. These water-soluble vitamins act as coenzymes in key metabolic pathways, especially those involving carbohydrates, fats, and protein metabolism. During menopause, many women report persistent fatigue, brain fog, and mood changes—symptoms directly tied to the functions B vitamins help regulate.

Vitamin B6 (pyridoxine) aids in the production of neurotransmitters such as serotonin and dopamine, which can influence mood and sleep patterns. Vitamin B9 (folate) is crucial for DNA repair and cellular renewal and plays a significant role in detoxifying excess estrogen metabolites through the liver. Vitamin B12 (cobalamin) is essential for the maintenance of the myelin sheath surrounding nerves and for red blood cell production, and its deficiency can mimic symptoms of dementia and cause fatigue and tingling in the extremities.

Together, B6, B9, and B12 help control levels of homocysteine, an amino acid that in excess can damage blood vessels and increase the risk of cardiovascular disease—a top concern during postmenopause. Since absorption of B12 decreases with age (especially in women with low stomach acid), supplementation or fortified foods may be required.

Symptom Relief and Prevention

- Support mental clarity and mood
- Reduce fatigue
- Aid estrogen metabolism through liver detox pathways
- Help reduce homocysteine, a cardiovascular risk factor

Recommended Intake

B6: 1.5 mg/day
B9 (folate): 400 mcg/day
B12: 2.4 mcg/day

Notable Food Sources of B Vitamins

Food	B Vitamin Content
Asparagus	134 mcg folate per ½ cup
Avocado	59 mcg folate per ½ fruit
Bananas	0.4 mg B6 per medium
Beef liver	70.7 mcg B12 per 3 oz
Black-eyed peas	105 mcg folate per ½ cup
Broccoli	104 mcg folate per cup
Brussels sprouts	78 mcg folate per cup

Food	B Vitamin Content
Chicken breast	0.5 mg B6 per 3 oz
Chickpeas	1.1 mg B6 per cup
Cottage cheese	0.2 mg B6 per cup
Eggs	0.6 mcg B12 per large
Fortified bread	60 mcg folate per slice
Fortified cereal	Amount per serving varies by brand
Lentils	358 mcg folate per cup
Milk	1.2 mcg B12 per cup
Nutritional yeast (fortified)	4 mcg B12 per tbsp
Oranges	55 mcg folate per medium
Potatoes	0.7 mg B6 per medium
Salmon	0.6 mg B6 per 3 oz
Spinach (cooked)	263 mcg folate per cup
Sunflower seeds	1.3 mg B6 per oz
Tempeh	0.2 mg B6 per ½ cup
Tofu	0.1 mg B6 per ½ cup
Tuna	2.5 mcg B12 per 3 oz
Yogurt	1.1 mcg B12 per cup

PHYTOESTROGENS: THE GENTLE HORMONE HELPERS

Why They Matter

Phytoestrogens are naturally occurring plant compounds that structurally resemble estrogen and can bind to estrogen receptors in the body. They have dual functionality based on the level of estrogen present. Though they are much weaker than the estrogen naturally made by the body, when the body is in a low-estrogen state they can have a balancing effect by imitating estrogen. When there is too much estrogen, they can block the activity of other compounds that try to increase the effects of estrogen. They can also block stronger xenoestrogens (external synthetic chemical compounds found in the environment that can mimic the body's natural estrogens and disrupt the endocrine system, potentially causing cancer, metabolic diseases like diabetes, and reproductive problems) or harmful estrogen metabolites (intermediate or end products of metabolism) when estrogen levels are already sufficient or too high.

In menopausal women, the body's natural estrogen production drops dramatically, leading to symptoms like hot flashes, night sweats, mood swings, and vaginal dryness. Phytoestrogens, especially isoflavones from soy and lignans from flaxseeds, can help gently modulate these symptoms by interacting with estrogen receptor beta (ERβ). This may have a protective, regulatory effect without overstimulating the system like hormone replacement therapy (HRT) can.

Beyond symptom management, phytoestrogens have been shown to improve lipid profiles, support bone density, and reduce the risk of hormone-dependent cancers such as breast and endometrial cancer. Their ability to lower inflammation and oxidative stress also makes them allies in the fight against aging.

Symptom Relief and Prevention

- Reduce hot flashes and night sweats
- Support bone and heart health
- Improve skin elasticity

Recommended Intake

Studies suggest 40–70 mg/day of isoflavones for symptom relief; however, there is no universal daily recommendation. This is optional based on your individual experience and needs.

Notable Food Sources of Phytoestrogens

Food	Phytoestrogen Type	Approximate Content
Alfalfa sprouts	Coumestans	0.5–1.5 mg per cup
Apples	Lignans	0.5–1 mg per medium
Barley (cooked)	Lignans	0.5–1.5 mg per cup
Black beans	Lignans	1.5–3 mg per cup
Bran cereal	Lignans	1–3 mg per cup
Carrots	Lignans	0.5 mg per medium
Chickpeas	Lignans	5–8 mg per cup
Edamame	Isoflavones	15 mg per ½ cup
Flaxseeds (ground)	Lignans	85–300 mg per 2 tbsp
Hummus	Lignans	3–5 mg per ¼ cup
Kidney beans	Lignans	1–2 mg per cup
Lentils	Lignans	2–4 mg per cup
Miso	Isoflavones	10–25 mg per tbsp
Mung beans	Lignans	1–2 mg per cup
Pumpkin seeds	Lignans	0.5–1.5 mg per oz
Red clover sprouts	Isoflavones	10–20 mg per cup
Rye bread	Lignans	0.8–1.2 mg per slice
Sesame seeds	Lignans	11–25 mg per tbsp
Soy milk	Isoflavones	6–10 mg per cup
Soy protein powder	Isoflavones	40–90 mg per scoop
Soybeans (cooked)	Isoflavones	20–25 mg per ½ cup
Sunflower seeds	Lignans	2–4 mg per oz
Tempeh	Isoflavones	35–60 mg per 3 oz
Tofu (firm)	Isoflavones	20–35 mg per 3 oz
Whole wheat bread	Lignans	0.5–1 mg per slice

VITAMIN E: THE SKIN AND NERVE SOOTHER

Why It Matters

Vitamin E is a fat-soluble antioxidant that protects cell membranes from oxidative damage. As oxidative stress increases with age—and particularly during menopause due to estrogen loss—vitamin E plays a vital role in preserving tissue health, neurological integrity, and immune defense.

One of its most specific benefits for menopausal women is the relief of vaginal dryness. Estrogen helps maintain the lubrication, elasticity, and thickness of vaginal tissues. Without it, the vaginal wall thins and becomes more fragile, increasing discomfort and risk of infection. Vitamin E, whether taken orally or used topically, can help restore moisture and reduce inflammation in vaginal tissue.

Vitamin E also protects nerve endings and may reduce the frequency and intensity of hot flashes when used in conjunction with omega-3 fatty acids. Furthermore, it improves skin appearance by enhancing wound healing, reducing hyperpigmentation, and promoting elasticity. Its anti-inflammatory and neuroprotective properties also make it valuable in protecting against age-related cognitive decline and cardiovascular damage.

Symptom Relief and Prevention

- Reduces vaginal dryness
- Helps with hot flashes (especially in combination with omega-3s)
- Supports eye and skin health

Recommended Intake

15 mg/day

Notable Food Sources of Vitamin E

Food	Vitamin E Content
Almonds	7.3 mg per oz
Apricots (dried)	1.5 mg per 10 halves
Asparagus	1.5 mg per cup
Avocado	2.1 mg per ½ fruit
Blackberries	1.0 mg per cup
Broccoli	1.2 mg per cup
Hazelnuts	4.3 mg per oz
Kale (cooked)	1.1 mg per cup
Kiwi	1.1 mg per fruit
Mango	1.5 mg per fruit
Mustard greens	1.8 mg per cup
Olive oil	1.9 mg per tbsp
Papaya	1.0 mg per cup
Peanut butter	2.9 mg per 2 tbsp
Pine nuts	2.6 mg per oz
Plant oils (sunflower/canola)	5–9 mg per tbsp
Pumpkin	1.3 mg per cup
Red bell pepper	1.9 mg per cup
Spinach (cooked)	3.7 mg per cup
Sunflower seeds	7.4 mg per oz
Swiss chard	3.3 mg per cup
Taro root	1.0 mg per cup
Tomato	0.7 mg per medium
Turnip greens	2.7 mg per cup
Wheat germ oil	20 mg per tbsp

ZINC: THE REPAIR MINERAL

Why It Matters

Zinc is a trace mineral involved in numerous enzymatic processes including wound healing, DNA synthesis, protein production, and immune function. During menopause, zinc becomes increasingly important for maintaining skin integrity, supporting immune response, and regulating hormonal activity.

Estrogen plays a role in skin hydration, elasticity, and collagen production. When levels fall, the skin often becomes thinner and more prone to dryness and sagging. Zinc supports the production of collagen and the repair of damaged skin tissue, making it essential for maintaining a youthful appearance and supporting healing. It's also critical for taste and smell, two senses that may change with age.

Zinc is heavily involved in immune modulation. Since immunity tends to weaken with age, adequate zinc intake is essential to reduce susceptibility to infections. It also influences libido and sexual health—areas often affected during menopause—by supporting vaginal tissue regeneration and sensitivity. Deficiency in zinc can lead to hair thinning, brittle nails, and delayed wound healing, all common concerns among menopausal women.

Symptom Relief and Prevention

- Boosts immune response
- May improve thinning hair and brittle nails
- Supports wound healing and skin health

Recommended Intake

8–12 mg/day

Notable Food Sources of Zinc

Food	Zinc Content
Almonds	0.9 mg per oz
Beef (grass-fed)	5.3 mg per 3 oz
Black beans	1.9 mg per cup
Cashews	1.6 mg per oz
Cheddar cheese	1.0 mg per oz
Chicken (dark meat)	2.7 mg per 3 oz
Chickpeas	2.5 mg per cup
Cocoa powder	1.9 mg per tbsp
Eggs	1.3 mg per 2 large
Green peas	1.2 mg per cup
Hemp seeds	2.0 mg per 3 tbsp
Lentils	2.5 mg per cup
Oats	2.3 mg per cup
Pine nuts	1.8 mg per oz
Pumpkin seeds	2.2 mg per oz
Quinoa	2.0 mg per cup
Shiitake mushrooms	1.0 mg per cup
Spinach (raw)	0.16 mg per cup
Sunflower seeds	1.5 mg per oz
Tahini	1.3 mg per tbsp
Tempeh	1.8 mg per ½ cup
Tofu	1.0 mg per ½ cup
Wheat germ	3.8 mg per oz
Yogurt	1.0 mg per cup

FOODS TO AVOID/LIMIT DURING MENOPAUSE

Just as some foods can be healing allies during the menopausal transition, others can work against your body's efforts to rebalance. Understanding what to avoid—or at least reduce—is just as important as knowing what to include. As estrogen levels decline, the body becomes more sensitive to certain foods that increase inflammation, disrupt blood sugar, interfere with sleep, or exacerbate symptoms like hot flashes, fatigue, mood swings, and weight gain.

Modern diets, often high in processed foods, added sugars, and synthetic additives, can significantly tax the body's systems already under strain during menopause. Many of these foods don't just offer "empty calories"—they actively contribute to hormonal disruption, metabolic dysfunction, and inflammation. For instance, excessive sugar not only contributes to insulin resistance but also increases the production of pro-inflammatory cytokines, which can worsen joint pain and hot flashes. Similarly, excessive alcohol, caffeine, and high-sodium foods can worsen night sweats, elevate blood pressure, and impair restful sleep.

In addition, the gut microbiome (the collection of microorganisms such as bacteria, fungi, and viruses that live in the gut), which is a key regulator of mood, weight, and immune function, is especially vulnerable during menopause. Artificial sweeteners, emulsifiers, and certain preservatives commonly found in ultra-processed foods can disrupt gut bacteria, leading to bloating, sluggish digestion, and even mental fog.

This section outlines a comprehensive list of foods that are best limited or avoided altogether during menopause. Each item is paired with a brief explanation of the potential harm or impact it may have on your physical and hormonal health. The goal is not rigid restriction but rather informed reduction. Many women find that simply becoming aware of these triggers and limiting or avoiding them can help reduce the frequency and severity of symptoms.

Small changes—swapping sweetened yogurt for plain Greek yogurt with berries, choosing whole-grain bread over white, or reducing processed snack consumption—can lead to meaningful improvements in energy, mood stability, and metabolic health. Remember, the quality of your nutrition directly affects the quality of your midlife experience. By removing the common dietary irritants and inflammatory agents outlined in the following chart, you free up the body's energy to heal, regulate, and thrive.

Foods to Limit or Avoid

Food/Ingredient	Reason to Limit/Avoid
Added sugars	Increase inflammation, blood sugar instability, and weight gain
Alcohol	Affects liver detox, sleep quality, and hormone metabolism
Artificial sweeteners	May disrupt gut microbiota and increase cravings
Caffeine	Triggers hot flashes, disrupts sleep
Charred meats	Can form carcinogenic compounds at high temperatures
Dairy (in some women)	Can worsen acne, inflammation, and joint pain
Energy drinks	Overstimulate the nervous system, disrupt sleep
Fast food	Typically high in unhealthy fats and low in nutrients
Flavored coffees	High in sugar, can trigger anxiety and night sweats
Fried foods	High in trans fats, promote oxidative stress
Granola bars	Often marketed as healthy but can be high in sugar, depending on the brand
High-sodium foods	Worsen bloating and blood pressure
Ice cream	High in sugar and dairy, may increase inflammation

Food/Ingredient	Reason to Limit/Avoid
Pastries and cakes	High in sugar and trans fats, poor nutrient density
Processed cheese	Contains additives, high in sodium
Processed meat (sausages, hot dogs)	High in nitrates and saturated fats
Processed snack foods	Often contain artificial additives and excess sodium
Red meat	Linked to increased cardiovascular and cancer risk
Refined carbohydrates	Cause insulin hormone spikes (which can lead to longer-term health problems such as weight gain, heart disease, kidney damage, and increased diabetes risk), fatigue, and increased belly fat
Sugary beverages	Cause rapid blood sugar spikes and crashes that can cause cravings, irritability, fatigue, and poor focus
Sweetened yogurts	Contain hidden sugars that can worsen hormonal balance
Trans fats	Promote inflammation and heart disease
White bread	Low in fiber, contributes to insulin resistance
White rice	Low in fiber, may spike blood sugar

3

LESS INFLAMMATION = EASIER MENOPAUSE

Menopause is frequently described as a hormonal roller coaster, but what often isn't mentioned is the underlying inflammation that fuels the most disruptive symptoms. Chronic, low-grade inflammation, sometimes referred to as "inflammaging," is not just a background process of aging, but a major player in the menopausal transition. This biological fire within can ignite everything from hot flashes and joint pain to mood swings and metabolic shifts. But what if the food on your plate could help extinguish that fire? Anti-inflammatory eating is more than just a wellness buzzword; it's a scientifically backed strategy that offers relief from menopausal symptoms while improving long-term health outcomes.

Estrogen and progesterone not only are key regulators of the reproductive cycle but also play crucial roles in the immune system, cardiovascular health, brain function, metabolism, and bone integrity. Estrogen, in particular, has known anti-inflammatory properties, so it makes sense that when estrogen levels drop dramatically during menopause, the balance can be tipped in favor of special chemicals called cytokines that can drive systemic inflammation throughout the body. This means that the very same changes that define menopause, hormonal shifts, also fuel the flames of internal inflammation.

The great news is that recent advances in nutritional science show us that what we eat can dramatically impact the body's inflammatory responses. Consuming an anti-inflammatory diet rich in whole, plant-based foods, omega-3 fats, antioxidants, and phytonutrients has been shown to lower circulating markers of inflammation such as C-reactive protein (CRP), interleukin-6 (IL-6), and tumor necrosis factor alpha (TNF-α). In the context of menopause, this anti-inflammatory dietary approach may ease the severity of vasomotor symptoms like hot flashes and night sweats, support cognitive function and mood stability, enhance sleep quality, and even help manage weight and cardiovascular risk.

Emerging studies support that women who adopt anti-inflammatory diets during menopause report better energy, fewer mood disturbances, reduced joint pain, and improved metabolic health. Moreover, these diets are protective in the long term—lowering the risk of osteoporosis, type 2 diabetes, cardiovascular disease, and cognitive decline. In essence, an anti-inflammatory diet isn't only beneficial for symptom management; it's also smart preventive medicine.

In the previous chapter we covered various critical nutrients that deserve special attention before, during, and after menopause. Building a solid anti-inflammatory style of eating involves increasing many of these nutrients while at the same time reducing or entirely eliminating inflammatory foods. You will notice that some of the nutrients discussed in the previous chapter can also be found in the chart that follows titled "Anti-Inflammatory Nutrient Quick Guide." This is not a mere coincidence. Those nutrients that need to be boosted during menopause also contribute to a reduced inflammatory environment within the body.

THE SCIENCE OF INFLAMMATION AND MENOPAUSE

Inflammation, when not in excess, is actually a critical part of how we survive as humans. It's a natural and vital part of the body's defense system, and without it, we would die. When you're injured or fighting off infection, your immune system deploys an army of white blood cells and chemical messengers to the affected area. Under normal circumstances, this acute inflammatory response is short-lived and helps the body heal. However, when inflammation becomes chronic—lasting weeks, months, or even years—it changes from a healing mechanism into a silent, destructive force that can damage tissues, organs, and systems throughout the body. In other words, there's a delicate balance the body must keep, as too much of a good thing can then become a bad thing.

Chronic inflammation is often invisible, yet it's the foundation of many of the most serious health issues of our time. Unlike acute inflammation, which causes obvious signs like redness or swelling, chronic inflammation may simmer beneath the surface without any outward symptoms. It can be triggered by a range of factors such as environmental toxins, chronic stress, unresolved infections, obesity, a sedentary lifestyle, and autoimmune activity (the immune system fighting against the body). Over time, this persistent immune activation exhausts the body's natural defenses and begins to disrupt normal function at every level.

One of the most serious consequences of chronic inflammation is its effect on the cardiovascular system. Inflammatory cells can accumulate in the walls of blood vessels, contributing to the formation of plaques that narrow the arteries in a process known as atherosclerosis. This can dramatically increase the risk of heart attack and stroke. A groundbreaking 2017 study in the *New England Journal of Medicine* led by Dr. Paul Ridker found that targeting inflammation with the drug canakinumab significantly reduced cardiovascular events in patients with a prior heart attack, even without altering cholesterol levels.[16] This research highlighted inflammation as a driving factor in heart disease independent of traditional risk factors.

Inflammation also poses a serious risk to brain health. Studies have linked chronic low-grade inflammation to a greater likelihood of neurodegenerative diseases such as Alzheimer's and Parkinson's. Additionally, pro-inflammatory cytokines like IL-6 and CRP have been associated with mood disorders, including depression and anxiety. One pivotal study based on the SWAN (Study of Women's Health Across the Nation) cohort revealed that even after adjusting for age, body mass index (BMI), and other lifestyle factors, postmenopausal women had elevated CRP and IL-6 levels—strong predictors of cardiovascular risk and systemic inflammation.[17] When the brain is under constant inflammatory assault, it may experience memory impairment, loss of focus, and diminished emotional regulation, thus essentially accelerating mental decline and increasing vulnerability to mental illness.

Menopause and Inflammation

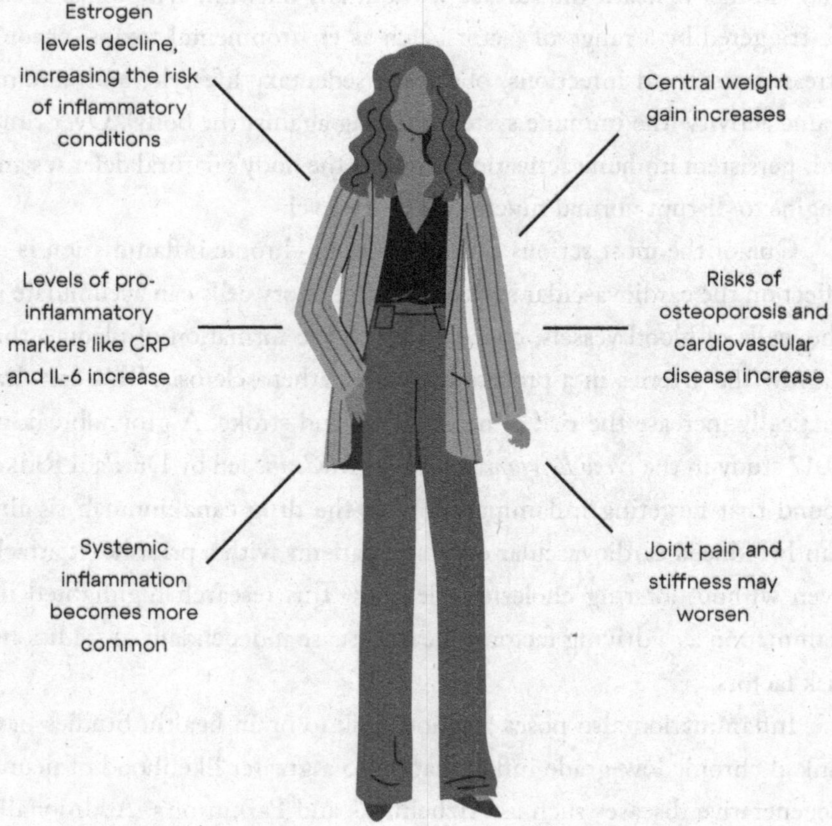

Ironically, the immune system becomes compromised when inflammation goes unchecked. While the immune system is designed to protect us, persistent inflammatory signaling can lead to autoimmune diseases like rheumatoid arthritis, lupus, and Hashimoto's thyroiditis, where the body mistakenly attacks its own healthy cells. At the same time, chronic inflammation that has gone unchecked for too long can actually weaken the immune response to real threats, making the body more susceptible to infections and even reducing its ability to identify and destroy cancerous cells.

Muscles and joints are another frequent casualty of chronic inflammation. Pro-inflammatory cytokines such as TNF-α, IL-1, and IL-6 play a direct role in breaking down joint cartilage and contributing to conditions like osteoarthritis and rheumatoid arthritis. Chronic inflammation also accelerates sarcopenia, the gradual loss of muscle mass and strength that occurs with aging. This muscle loss can lead to decreased mobility, increased risk of falls, and a reduced ability to perform everyday tasks.

On a metabolic level, inflammation interferes with insulin signaling, contributing to insulin resistance and the development of type 2 diabetes. Adipose (fat) tissue, especially visceral fat stored around the organs, can become inflamed and secrete additional cytokines, creating a vicious cycle of weight gain and metabolic dysfunction. Obesity itself is both a cause and consequence of chronic inflammation, further complicating efforts to achieve metabolic health.

The digestive system can also suffer. Chronic inflammation can compromise the integrity of the intestinal lining, leading to increased intestinal permeability, or what's commonly known as "leaky gut." This allows toxins and undigested food particles to escape into the bloodstream, provoking further immune responses. Conditions like irritable bowel syndrome (IBS), Crohn's disease, and ulcerative colitis are all linked to chronic inflammation of the gut. Moreover, disruptions to the gut microbiome—our internal ecosystem of beneficial microorganisms such as bacteria, viruses, and fungi—can both contribute to and be worsened by inflammation.

In the realm of hormonal health, chronic inflammation can throw key systems into disarray. It has been shown to interfere with the body's estrogen and progesterone receptors, which can exacerbate menstrual irregularities, intensify menopause symptoms, and impair fertility. It can also dysregulate cortisol, the primary hormone that responds to stress, leading to symptoms such as fatigue, poor sleep, and mood instability. Women in midlife, especially during perimenopause and menopause, when hormones are already fluctuating, may be particularly vulnerable to inflammation-induced hormonal shifts.

Perhaps most alarmingly, chronic inflammation lays the groundwork for cancer. Long-term inflammation can damage the DNA in our cells, promote unchecked cell growth, and suppress the body's natural ability to detect and fight tumors. It's well-documented that certain chronic inflammatory conditions increase cancer risk. For example, hepatitis can cause liver cancer, inflammatory bowel diseases have been linked to colorectal cancer, and chronic gastritis may lead to stomach cancer. In these cases, inflammation not only acts as a trigger, but also promotes tumor growth and progression.

The symptoms of chronic inflammation are often subtle but can be telling. They include ongoing fatigue, unexplained weight gain, brain fog, joint or muscle pain, digestive discomfort, skin breakouts, and frequent infections. These signals are often dismissed or misattributed to aging or stress, when they may actually be early warnings of deeper inflammation at work.

The hormonal fluctuations of menopause—especially the dramatic drop in estrogen—fundamentally alter the body's inflammatory landscape. Estrogen binds to immune cells, prompting them to carry out their important work of lowering inflammation. Declining estrogen levels mean less activation of these immune cells and a decreased ability to reduce inflammation.

A 2021 study in the *Journal of Clinical Psychiatry* looking at menopause, inflammation, and depression found that elevated inflammatory markers during menopause were associated with increased risk for depressive symptoms, regardless of age or BMI.[18] This underscores the systemic impact of inflammation during this life phase—not just physically, but emotionally and neurologically as well.

The encouraging news is that, while some level of inflammation is inevitable with aging, its intensity and impact can be influenced by the choices we make every day. Through regular movement, stress management, quality sleep, reduced exposure to toxins, and especially proper nutrition, we can begin to calm this internal fire. Anti-inflammatory diets, such as the Mediterranean or DASH diets, have proven effective in lowering systemic inflammation. Anti-inflammatory foods rich in antioxidants, fiber, omega-3s, and polyphenols (like leafy greens, berries, olive oil, turmeric, and fatty fish) help counteract inflammatory processes. Meanwhile, avoiding ultra-processed foods, trans fats, smoking, and excessive sugar can also reduce inflammatory triggers. Anti-inflammatory nutrition offers a protective strategy, one that can buffer against the harsh physiological changes of menopause while improving quality of life.

Understanding this science transforms the conversation around menopause. Rather than viewing inflammation as an unavoidable burden of aging, we can begin to see it as a modifiable process, one that responds to the foods we choose, how we manage stress, the way we move, and how well we sleep. With the right tools and knowledge, menopause can become a powerful opportunity to reset, rebuild, and rejuvenate.

UNDERSTANDING AN ANTI-INFLAMMATORY DIET

An anti-inflammatory diet is a nutritional approach that focuses on reducing chronic inflammation in the body. The goal is to shift the body into a more balanced, resilient state by nourishing it with foods that help calm inflammation. The foundation of an anti-inflammatory diet includes a wide variety of whole, plant-based foods, rich in vitamins, minerals, fiber, and antioxidants. These include colorful fruits and vegetables—particularly those high in flavonoids and polyphenols, like berries, leafy greens, cruciferous vegetables, and bell peppers—which contain fiber and antioxidants that help neutralize the dangerous compounds called free radicals that are responsible for oxidative stress. Whole grains like quinoa, brown rice, and oats provide fiber to support gut health, which is intimately connected to inflammation control. Legumes, beans, nuts, and seeds offer plant-based protein and healthy fats, while fatty fish such as salmon, sardines, and mackerel deliver essential omega-3 fatty acids known for their strong anti-inflammatory effects.

Another key aspect of this diet is the use of anti-inflammatory herbs and spices. Turmeric, which contains curcumin, is one of the most powerful anti-inflammatory compounds studied, while ginger, garlic, cinnamon, and rosemary also provide potent bioactive compounds that support immune regulation and reduce inflammation. Olive oil, especially extra-virgin olive oil, is a rich source of healthy monounsaturated fats and polyphenols. Avocados, flaxseeds, chia seeds, and walnuts are additional healthy fat sources that contribute to reducing inflammation and supporting heart and brain health.

We often talk about what to consume in an anti-inflammatory diet, but what is equally important is understanding what to *exclude.* An important goal is to minimize or avoid processed and refined foods, such as white bread, sugary snacks, and sweetened beverages, which can spike blood sugar and promote inflammatory pathways. Red and processed meats, trans fats, and excessive alcohol consumption are also discouraged, as they have been shown to increase markers of inflammation in the body. Instead, the emphasis is on mindful, intentional eating that supports energy, hormonal balance, and cellular repair.

Overall, an anti-inflammatory diet is not a short-term fix, but rather a long-term lifestyle approach. It is not about strict rules, perfection, or deprivation, but about consistently choosing foods that fuel the body, support healthy aging, and reduce the risk of chronic disease. Many people who follow this type of diet, regardless of age, report improved energy levels, clearer skin, better digestion, reduced joint pain, and enhanced mental clarity when adopting this way of eating. Its benefits go beyond inflammation control as it fosters resilience, wellness, and a deeper connection to food as medicine.

The following tables list key anti-inflammatory nutrients, with at least ten food sources for each, and key anti-inflammatory foods, offering dietary guidance for managing menopause-related inflammation and supporting overall health. You will see some overlap, but I wanted to include both charts for your ease of use.

Anti-Inflammatory Nutrient Quick Guide

Nutrient	Top 10 Food Sources
Calcium	Almonds, Sardines, Kale, Yogurt, Tofu, Broccoli, Chia seeds, Fortified plant milks, Okra, Bok choy
Fiber	Oats, Lentils, Chickpeas, Black beans, Pears, Apples, Broccoli, Carrots, Chia seeds, Whole grains
Folate	Lentils, Spinach, Asparagus, Broccoli, Avocado, Oranges, Peas, Beets, Chickpeas, Fortified cereals
Magnesium	Spinach, Pumpkin seeds, Almonds, Black beans, Avocado, Dark chocolate, Quinoa, Bananas, Cashews, Tofu
Omega-3 Fatty Acids	Salmon, Sardines, Mackerel, Tuna, Herring, Oysters, Chia seeds, Flaxseeds, Walnuts, Hemp seeds, Cod-liver oil, Soybeans, Seaweed
Polyphenols	Berries, Green tea, Dark chocolate, Olives, Apples, Red grapes, Citrus fruits, Turmeric, Coffee, Artichokes
Tryptophan	Pumpkin seeds, Turkey, Oats, Soybeans, Eggs, Tofu, Cheese, Sesame seeds, Chicken breast, Peanuts
Vitamin B6	Bananas, Sunflower seeds, Spinach, Salmon, Chicken, Tuna, Avocado, Turkey, Sweet potatoes, Fortified cereals
Vitamin C	Bell peppers, Oranges, Strawberries, Kiwi, Broccoli, Brussels sprouts, Pineapple, Mango, Papaya, Tomatoes
Vitamin K	Kale, Spinach, Broccoli, Brussels sprouts, Parsley, Natto, Green beans, Cabbage, Prunes, Asparagus

Anti-Inflammatory Food Quick Guide

Food	Nutrients	Benefits
Beets	Betalains, nitrates	Support vascular health and reduce inflammation markers
Berries	Anthocyanins, vitamin C	Protect against cellular damage
Fatty fish (mackerel, salmon, sardines)	Omega-3s	Reduce inflammation and support heart/brain health
Flaxseeds	Lignans, ALA	Balance estrogen levels and fight inflammation
Ginger	Gingerol	Relieves joint pain and improves digestion
Green tea	Epigallocatechin gallate (EGCG)	Reduces inflammation and enhances metabolism
Leafy greens	Magnesium, vitamin K	Support bones, mood, and immune health
Legumes	Fiber, protein	Support blood sugar balance and gut health
Nuts (almonds, walnuts)	Omega-3s, vitamin E	Protect the brain and heart and reduce oxidative stress
Olive oil	Polyphenols	Improves heart health and lowers inflammatory markers
Pineapple	Bromelain	Reduces inflammation and improves digestion
Red cabbage	Anthocyanins, vitamin C	Protects against cellular damage
Turmeric	Curcumin	Inhibits pro-inflammatory cytokines

TARGETED RELIEF THROUGH ANTI-INFLAMMATORY EATING

Anti-inflammatory foods and nutrients have been shown through vast research to have true physiological impact within the body. Some of these nutrients that we can get through food have been extracted, synthesized, and concentrated into supplements. In most cases, however, natural food sources make the nutrients more available to the body for absorption and use. If you are not getting enough through your diet, properly screened and verified supplements can be a helpful addition.

- **Bone health:** Menopause accelerates bone turnover, leading to a rapid decline in bone mineral density (BMD), particularly in the first five years postmenopause. Chronic inflammation exacerbates this loss by promoting the further breakdown of bone tissue. Magnesium (pumpkin seeds and spinach), vitamin K (kale and fermented foods), and calcium (almonds and fortified plant milks) all play vital roles in bone preservation. Additionally, omega-3 fatty acids help suppress cytokines that promote bone loss. Studies indicate that postmenopausal women with higher intakes of anti-inflammatory nutrients have better BMD scores and reduced fracture risk.[19]
- **Cardiovascular health:** With the decline of estrogen, women face increased cardiovascular risks, including hypertension, atherosclerosis, and dyslipidemia (abnormal level of lipids in the blood). Anti-inflammatory diets rich in monounsaturated fats (olive oil, avocados), omega-3s, fiber, and flavonoids (berries, leafy greens, chocolate, soybeans) help reduce oxidative stress and prevent plaque buildup in arteries. Anti-inflammatory diets improve the function of the cells lining our blood vessels and lower LDL cholesterol. A comprehensive meta-analysis confirmed that adherence

to a Mediterranean-style diet significantly reduces cardiovascular mortality and events.[20]

- **Hot flashes and night sweats:** Vasomotor symptoms like hot flashes and night sweats are among the most reported complaints during menopause, affecting up to 75 percent of women. These are triggered by the hypothalamus's (the body's master control center) altered response to slight changes in body temperature due to declining estrogen. Omega-3 fatty acids, particularly from cold-water fish like salmon and plant-based sources like flaxseeds and chia seeds, are known to reduce inflammation and stabilize neurotransmitter pathways related to thermoregulation. Anti-inflammatory compounds may also help balance prostaglandins, chemical messengers involved in temperature control. While more studies are ongoing, a randomized controlled trial published in the journal *Menopause* showed that omega-3 supplementation significantly reduced the frequency and severity of hot flashes.[21]
- **Mood, anxiety, and cognitive health:** Mood disorders often intensify during the menopausal transition, with declining estrogen disrupting neurotransmitter systems such as serotonin, dopamine, and GABA. Anti-inflammatory diets that are rich in omega-3s (walnuts, flaxseeds, fatty fish), folate (leafy greens, beans), and polyphenols (berries, olive oil) may reduce neuroinflammation and oxidative stress—two major contributors to mood dysregulation and cognitive decline. Regular consumption of these nutrients has been shown to lower the incidence of depression. Furthermore, high-antioxidant foods may preserve hippocampal volume, supporting memory and executive function.[22]
- **Sleep quality:** Sleep disturbances affect over 60 percent of menopausal women, often due to a combination of hormonal changes, night sweats, and mood disorders. An anti-inflammatory diet supports better sleep by providing nutrients that enhance the production of serotonin and melatonin. Tryptophan (oats, seeds, poultry),

magnesium (leafy greens, legumes), and vitamin B6 (bananas, avocados) are involved in calming the nervous system. Chronic inflammation interferes with the circadian rhythms that help regulate sleep, so reducing it through diet can help restore proper sleep cycles. One study found that women with high inflammatory diets were more likely to suffer from poor sleep and insomnia.[23]

- **Weight and blood sugar regulation:** Weight gain—especially in the abdominal area—is a hallmark of the menopausal transition. Visceral fat increases systemic inflammation, perpetuating a cycle of insulin resistance and metabolic dysfunction. An anti-inflammatory diet rich in fiber, omega-3s, and phytonutrients helps regulate insulin response and reduce fasting glucose levels. Whole grains, lentils, cruciferous vegetables, and berries improve metabolic flexibility.

BEWARE OF INFLAMMATORY FOODS

Just as incorporating anti-inflammatory foods can support hormonal health and symptom relief, minimizing or eliminating pro-inflammatory foods is equally important. Diets high in refined sugars, trans fats, processed meats, and highly processed packaged foods have been shown to increase systemic inflammation, exacerbate hot flashes, disrupt sleep, and contribute to weight gain and mood instability. During menopause, the body's resilience to these stressors is diminished, making it even more critical to adopt a nutrient-dense, whole-food-based approach to eating. By reducing inflammatory triggers, women can help regulate hormonal fluctuations, protect cardiovascular and bone health, and improve overall quality of life.

You'll notice the following list intentionally overlaps with the list of foods to avoid during menopause that was located in chapter two. The reason these foods should be avoided is largely because of their inflammatory properties.

Foods to Avoid for Inflammation Management

Food	Reason to Avoid
Alcohol (in excess)	Damages the liver and disrupts hormone balance
Artificial sweeteners	Alter gut microbiota and may promote inflammation
Fried foods (chips, fried chicken)	Contain trans fats, which raise "bad" cholesterol (LDL) and lower "good" cholesterol (HDL), and AGEs (advanced glycation end products), which contribute to inflammation, oxidative stress, and chronic diseases like heart disease, kidney disease, and diabetes
Highly processed snacks	Low in nutrients, high in sugar/salt/fats
Processed meats (bacon, sausage)	Contain nitrates and pro-inflammatory compounds
Refined carbs (white bread, pastries)	Increase blood sugar and CRP levels
Sugary beverages (soda, juices)	Promote insulin resistance and inflammation

THE ANTI-INFLAMMATORY LIFESTYLE

Adopting anti-inflammatory lifestyle habits beyond nutrition can play a critical role in managing menopausal symptoms and promoting overall well-being. These strategies support hormonal balance, reduce oxidative stress, and help buffer the effects of aging on key systems such as the cardiovascular, nervous, and immune systems.

- **Exercise:** Engaging in regular, moderate physical activity such as walking, strength training, or swimming helps reduce systemic inflammation by lowering CRP levels and increasing the production of anti-inflammatory cytokines. Exercise also improves mood, bone density, and insulin sensitivity, making it a cornerstone of menopausal wellness.

- **Gut health:** A balanced gut microbiome plays a central role in immune response modulation and inflammation control. Including fermented foods like yogurt, kefir, kimchi, and sauerkraut—as well as prebiotic fibers from foods like onions, garlic, bananas, and oats—supports microbial diversity. This, in turn, helps regulate estrogen metabolism and contributes to reduced inflammation levels system wide.
- **Sleep hygiene:** Sleep is essential for hormonal recovery and immune regulation. Poor sleep—especially when fragmented or under six hours a night—can elevate pro-inflammatory markers such as IL-6 and TNF-α. Creating a sleep-supportive environment, maintaining a consistent bedtime, and avoiding screen use close to bedtime can help women achieve the seven to nine hours of restful sleep needed for recovery and hormone regulation.
- **Stress management:** Chronic stress leads to elevated cortisol levels that can promote inflammation and disrupt hormone balance. Mindfulness practices, yoga, guided breathing, and journaling have all been shown to calm the nervous system, reduce stress biomarkers, and improve emotional resilience during menopause.

NOURISHING YOUR SECOND ACT

Inflammation is an important protective responsive for the body, and in proper amounts it's critical for overall health and protection at all times throughout our life. However, too much inflammation and our bodies suffer. Chronic inflammation can be brought on by many factors, some of which are not in our direct control (autoimmune disorders, genetic factors, our environment). However, the foods we consume *are* within our control and selecting which to increase in our diets and which to reduce or eliminate can be an important part of reducing inflammation.

The menopausal transition is not merely a biological event, but a holistic, multifaceted journey that affects every aspect of a woman's life. While its symptoms and health implications can be challenging, menopause also offers an opportunity for personal renewal and empowerment. By embracing evidence-based strategies such as anti-inflammatory nutrition, lifestyle modifications, stress reduction, and integrative therapies, women can actively shape their health and vitality in this new chapter.

As cliché as it might sound, knowledge is definitely power, and understanding the physiological changes behind menopause provides the foundation for making informed choices. Women deserve more than to suffer in silence; they deserve accurate information, compassionate care, and the freedom to thrive through menopause and beyond.

Menopause should not be viewed as the end, because it's a new beginning rich with opportunity to reclaim vitality. Food becomes a tool not just for symptom relief but for total body transformation. By embracing an anti-inflammatory way of eating, women can regain control over their bodies, their minds, and their futures. This is a journey of empowerment, one day and one plate at a time. The choices that are made aggregate and compound over time, making daily nourishment a declaration that thriving is not behind you but ahead. It is possible to age with strength, clarity, and the joy of knowing that wellness is still within reach—deliciously, sustainably, and powerfully. The meal plan in the next chapter incorporates an anti-inflammatory approach as well as other strategies that will help alleviate symptoms, promote weight loss, and improve overall wellness.

4

THE NEW MENOPAUSE KITCHEN MEAL PLAN

The focus of this ten-week meal plan is on nutrient-rich foods that help alleviate menopausal symptoms like hot flashes, weight gain, and mood changes. It includes foods high in fiber, phytoestrogens, healthy fats, calcium, and other nutrients. These snacks and meals are simple enough to be made without recipes, though options are offered from the recipes in appendix I, and they are full of ingredients that are known to help alleviate menopausal symptoms, reduce inflammation, and support overall health. You might not like all of the foods on the plan, so I have given you options at the end of each week that you can substitute into the meal plan to suit your palate preference and budget.

This plan was designed to incorporate as many of the power nutrients mentioned in chapter two as possible. While this is not a classically low-calorie diet, it is what I call a "smart-calorie" diet. The calorie count for each day falls well below 2,000 (usually between 1,200 and 1,400), but more importantly, these calories come with lots of nutrients that have significant health benefits. Feel free to make as many substitutions as you like, but make sure those substitutions follow the General Guidelines on page 72. Your substitutions should follow a similar nutrient profile. For example, don't substitute steak or fish for a salad.

The weeks are specifically designed to maximize results, so the order in which you follow them is important. Don't skip around the weeks, but do your best to follow them as they are written. However, I have created many alternate meal options so that you're not eating the same foods all the time. The more diverse your choices, the less likely you are to drift away from the program due to "food fatigue." Food boredom is a major reason people do not comply with their meal programs. You will find different options for different weeks, and this is not random. The weeks and days have different nutrient and calorie profiles, so the options have been selected to fit that day or week. You can also make use of the recipes and snacks in the back of the book as additional options when you want to try something different. They were created so that you could try new food combinations and flavors and still get the nutrients that will be helpful.

Hundreds of women have tried this plan and found great success. While the individual results varied, many reported significant weight loss, a noticeable reduction in some of their menopausal symptoms, improved waistline measurements, and increased energy. You will meet some of these women and their amazing success stories in chapter six. None of those women were perfect when following the plan, and you don't have to be either. I've written the program with that in mind. I expect you to have bad days or even a bad week. I also don't expect you to cook every meal at home under tight dietary restrictions. That would be onerous and unrealistic for most. I expect you to sometimes go out to a restaurant or order takeout. That is completely fine. Just remember, when you are getting your food from another source, use the meal in the plan as a guideline for the type and quantity of food that you order. For example, if your meal plan dinner options are fish and vegetables, try to stick to those general categories when eating out and don't order something like pizza instead.

I chose ten weeks because that is a long enough time for most people to notice benefits and so that it offers sufficient variety for the future. Once you have completed the ten-week program, you can take a small break and then try another round, or you can break up the program into two-week or three-week intervals and do them as often as you like, prioritizing the weeks you like best. You can even make up your own plan by using the recipes and snacks in the back of the book. If you decide to do this, make sure when you choose the weeks that you do them in chronological order. For example, if you choose weeks 3, 5, and 7, do them in that order. Don't do week 7, then 3 and 5.

The idea is that after completing the first ten weeks, you'll be able to use your experience as a guideline for what to do in the future. Take note of what worked and what didn't so that, when you want to re-engage with the plan, you can avoid previous mistakes and challenges and focus on what worked and brought you the best results. Feel free to modify and adapt the plan so that it fits you. The goal is not for you to be on a strict meal plan forever, but rather to teach you sound nutritional strategies so you can make changes to your diet that are enjoyable and sustainable and become part of your daily life.

Most importantly, open your mind and palate and try different foods. You might be surprised by what you actually like. Bon appétit!

General Guidelines

- Drink plenty of water. If you want something other than water, try unsweetened herbal tea.
- Include a variety of fruits and vegetables to maximize nutrient intake.
- Aim for regularly timed meals to stabilize blood sugar and manage weight.
- If you don't like or can't access the foods specified for a certain day, choose an alternate day from the options at the end of each week. Make sure you are substituting from the specified options list based on the day of the week you are substituting for.
- Any snack listed can be swapped out and replaced with a smoothie that is 200 calories or less.
- Feel free to make fruit substitutions. For example, if the meal plan calls for pineapples and you don't like or have them, substitute berries or another fruit.
- If you don't like the fish listed for that day's menu, substitute another fish of your choice. Try to grill or bake your fish rather than fry it.
- Any lunch or dinner in the meal plan can be replaced by 1½ cups of soup, such as tomato, mixed vegetable, miso, lentil, pea, squash, carrot, cabbage, black bean, cauliflower, broccoli, or chicken and vegetable. Look for low-sodium options.
- Salads should be a total of 2 to 3 cups for all ingredients combined.
- Yogurt servings should be approximately 5 ounces. Choose nonfat, low-fat, or 2 percent fat, with 3 grams or less of added sugars (look for the word "unsweetened" on the label, as that typically keeps the sugar content low).
- When selecting a peanut butter or almond butter, make sure the sugar content is 2 grams or less per 2-tablespoon serving.
- Limit added sugars, refined carbs, and processed foods.

- Limit Brazil nuts to 1 to 3 per day maximum to avoid excess selenium ingestion.
- On resistance/strength training days (see chapter five), increase protein intake in your snacks and meals by 30 percent.

WEEK 1

Day 1

Breakfast: ¾ cup Greek yogurt with ¼ cup walnuts

Lunch: Quinoa salad with kale, chickpeas, avocado, and light lemon-tahini dressing

Dinner: Lentil and vegetable stew with carrots, celery, and tomatoes (or try the Lentil and Spinach Soup recipe on page 218)

Day 2

Breakfast: Apple slices with 2 tablespoons almond or other nut butter

Lunch: Mixed greens salad with chickpeas, cherry tomatoes, cucumber, and light lemon–olive oil dressing

Snack: 10 to 12 raw almonds

Dinner: Baked or grilled salmon (6 ounces) with steamed asparagus, ½ cup quinoa, and mixed greens (or try the Baked Salmon with Asparagus recipe on page 198)

Day 3

Breakfast: 1 cup mixed fruit with 2 tablespoons low-fat cottage cheese

Lunch: Mixed greens salad with roasted sweet potatoes, beets, goat cheese, and light balsamic vinaigrette dressing

Dinner: Stir-fry with tofu (6 ounces), broccoli, bell peppers, and sesame-ginger sauce (optional: substitute brown or purple rice for the tofu)

Day 4

Breakfast: 2 scrambled eggs with diced vegetables

Lunch: Lentil soup with slice of whole-grain bread

Snack: 1 orange

Dinner: Stir-fry with salmon or chicken (6 ounces), broccoli, bell peppers, and snap peas over ½ cup brown rice

Day 5

Breakfast: 1 cup blueberries with 2 tablespoons Greek yogurt

Lunch: Mediterranean tuna salad with cucumber, cherry tomatoes, red onion, olives, and feta cheese (or try the Mediterranean Orzo Salad recipe on page 223)

Dinner: Baked bell peppers stuffed with quinoa, black beans, corn, and shredded cheese (optional: substitute brown or purple rice for the quinoa)

Day 6

Breakfast: Banana with 2 tablespoons peanut butter

Lunch: Spinach and feta salad with walnuts, dried cranberries, and light balsamic vinaigrette dressing

Snack: Carrot sticks with 2 tablespoons hummus

Dinner: Grilled chicken breast (4 ounces) with roasted sweet potatoes and Brussels sprouts

Day 7

Breakfast: 1 cup mixed berries with 2 tablespoons Greek yogurt (or make it a smoothie with 1 cup berries and ½ cup low-fat milk)

Lunch: Spinach and arugula salad with roasted butternut squash, walnuts, and light vinaigrette dressing

Dinner: Eggplant and zucchini bake with tomato sauce and mozzarella cheese (or try the Zucchini Noodles with Pesto and Cherry Tomatoes recipe on page 248)

Alternate Options
Odd Days

Choose any of the following options to substitute into the main program for odd days only.

Option 1

Breakfast: 1 cup mixed diced melon with 2 tablespoons low-fat cottage cheese

Lunch: Arugula and mixed greens salad with roasted asparagus, raw sunflower seeds, and light lemon vinaigrette dressing

Dinner: Baked acorn squash filled with quinoa, apple, and cinnamon

Option 2

Breakfast: 1 cup warm or cold fortified cereal with milk

Lunch: Spinach salad with roasted red onion, goat cheese, walnuts, and light balsamic dressing

Dinner: Vegetable soup with kale, chickpeas, and carrots, and slice of whole-grain bread

Option 3

Breakfast: Protein shake or smoothie (12 ounces) 300 calories or less

Lunch: Mediterranean bulgur salad with tomatoes, cucumbers, parsley, and light lemon–olive oil dressing

Dinner: Stir-fry with tofu (6 ounces), green beans, shiitake mushrooms, and ginger-garlic sauce

Option 4

Breakfast: 1 cup diced mango with a squeeze of lime

Lunch: Mixed greens salad with artichoke hearts, roasted red peppers, raw sunflower seeds, and light lemon-tahini dressing

Dinner: Baked portobello mushroom cap stuffed with lentils, spinach, and feta cheese

Option 5

Breakfast: 2 scrambled eggs and slice of whole-grain toast topped with ½ mashed avocado

Lunch: Arugula salad with roasted butternut squash, dried cranberries, raw pecans, and light balsamic vinaigrette dressing

Dinner: Stir-fry with tofu (6 ounces), bell peppers, cauliflower rice, and sesame-tamari sauce

Option 6

Breakfast: ¼ cup Greek yogurt with ¼ cup low-sugar granola and blueberries

Lunch: Spinach and arugula salad with roasted sweet potatoes, chickpeas, and ½ avocado

Dinner: Baked bell peppers stuffed with farro, black beans, corn, and shredded cheese

Even Days

Choose any of the following options to substitute into the main program for even days only.

Option 1

Breakfast: Apple slices with 2 tablespoons hazelnut butter

Lunch: Roasted vegetable and lentil bowl with red bell pepper, eggplant, and kale

Snack: ½ cup pineapple chunks

Dinner: Grilled lamb chop (6 ounces) with roasted Brussels sprouts and mashed parsnips

Option 2

Breakfast: ¾ cup Greek yogurt with 1 tablespoon chia seeds and blueberries

Lunch: Barley and chickpea salad with carrots, celery, and light lemon-tahini dressing

Snack: 1 plum

Dinner: Baked flounder (6 ounces) with roasted sweet potato fries and sautéed spinach

Option 3

Breakfast: 1 cup papaya, mango, and kiwi slices with ½ cup low-fat cottage cheese

Lunch: Shredded cabbage and carrot slaw with sesame seeds, tofu strips, and light ginger-soy dressing

Snack: 1 hard-boiled egg

Dinner: Grilled chicken or turkey burger (4 ounces) with roasted rainbow carrots and steamed green beans

Option 4

Breakfast: ½ cup low-fat ricotta with honey drizzle and strawberries

Lunch: Freekeh salad with roasted red peppers, chickpeas, chopped cucumber, and light herb dressing

Snack: ½ cup edamame

Dinner: Baked swordfish (4 ounces) with sautéed kale and quinoa

Option 5

Snack: ½ cup low-fat cottage cheese with strawberries

Lunch: Warm quinoa bowl with roasted sweet potato, black beans, corn, ½ avocado, and light lime dressing

Snack: 1 apple

Dinner: Grilled skinless turkey or chicken breast (6 ounces) with roasted cauliflower and wild rice

Option 6

Snack: Banana with 2 tablespoons almond or peanut butter

Lunch: Mixed greens salad with olives, artichoke hearts, red onion, and light lemon–olive oil dressing

Snack: Cucumber slices with 2 tablespoons hummus

Dinner: Grilled sea bass (4 ounces) with roasted parsnips and steamed broccoli

WEEK 2

Day 1

Breakfast: 2 banana protein pancakes with light syrup

Lunch: Lentil salad with diced cucumbers, red bell peppers, red onion, and light lemon–olive oil dressing (or try the Quinoa and Black Bean Salad recipe on page 231)

Dinner: Cauliflower and chickpea curry with coconut milk over ½ cup brown rice

Day 2

Breakfast: 1 cup mixed berries with 2 tablespoons Greek yogurt (or try the Almond Butter and Banana Smoothie recipe on page 186)

Lunch: Chickpea and avocado salad with cherry tomatoes, cucumber, and olive oil

Snack: ¼ cup walnut halves

Dinner: Baked cod (6 ounces) with sautéed kale and ½ cup wild rice

Day 3

Breakfast: Slice of whole-grain toast with 1 scrambled egg and ½ avocado

Lunch: Kale salad with roasted chickpeas, avocado, pumpkin seeds, and light turmeric dressing (optional: substitute other greens for the kale) (or try the Roasted Sweet Potato and Chickpea Bowl recipe on page 234)

Dinner: Baked portobello mushroom cap stuffed with quinoa, spinach, and sun-dried tomatoes

Day 4

Breakfast: 1 cup oatmeal, cooked, with apple chunks, cinnamon, and walnuts

Lunch: Mixed bean salad with bell peppers, red onion, parsley, and light lemon–olive oil dressing

Snack: Cucumber slices with 2 tablespoons tzatziki

Dinner: Grilled turkey burger (6 ounces, no bun) with roasted carrots and green beans

Day 5

Breakfast: Veggie breakfast quesadilla with 2 eggs, low-fat cheese, and bell peppers in a whole-grain tortilla

Lunch: Warm quinoa bowl with roasted zucchini, eggplant, bell peppers, and tahini drizzle (optional: substitute another grain like rice, sorghum, bulgur, etc. for the quinoa)

Dinner: Stir-fry with shrimp (6 medium), mixed vegetables, and cauliflower rice (or try the Cauliflower Rice Stir-Fry recipe on page 201)

Day 6

Breakfast: Smoothie (12 ounces) with 1½ cups coconut water, 25 grams protein powder, ½ cup mango, and ½ cup raw spinach

Lunch: Roasted vegetable salad with carrots, bell peppers, red onion, and tahini sauce (or try the Spicy Hummus with Veggies recipe on page 235)

Snack: 1 kiwi or other piece of fruit

Dinner: Stir-fry with tofu (6 ounces), snap peas, mushrooms, and garlic-soy sauce (optional: substitute ½ cup diced chicken for the tofu)

Day 7

Breakfast: Slice of whole-grain toast topped with 2 tablespoons low-fat cottage cheese and sliced tomato

Lunch: Mediterranean salad with mixed greens, olives, cucumber, feta cheese, and light vinaigrette dressing

Dinner: Baked chicken thigh (4 ounces) with roasted butternut squash and steamed broccoli

Alternate Options
Odd Days

Choose any of the following options to substitute into the main program for odd days only.

Option 1

Breakfast: Peanut butter–banana overnight oats with 1½ cups low-fat milk, 1 cup whole oats, 1 tablespoon peanut butter, and ½ small banana, sliced, put in a jar and refrigerated overnight

Lunch: Farro salad with roasted red peppers, olives, arugula, and light lemon-tahini dressing

Dinner: Roasted eggplant stuffed with lentils, tomatoes, and fresh basil

Option 2

Breakfast: Breakfast bowl with ½ cup brown rice, 1 scrambled egg, and ½ avocado, sliced

Lunch: Mixed greens salad with roasted butternut squash, edamame, walnuts, and light balsamic dressing

Dinner: Cauliflower and chickpea curry served over ½ cup quinoa

Option 3

Breakfast: High-fiber, low-sugar cereal with low-fat milk and sliced banana

Lunch: Roasted beet and goat cheese salad with spinach, pumpkin seeds, and light lemon vinaigrette dressing

Dinner: Zucchini fritters with mixed greens and light tahini sauce

Option 4

Breakfast: ½ cup low-fat cottage cheese with apple slices and cinnamon

Lunch: Tabbouleh with quinoa, parsley, diced tomatoes, cucumber, and light lemon–olive oil dressing

Dinner: Baked acorn squash filled with black beans, kale, and feta cheese

Option 5

Breakfast: Veggie scramble with 2 eggs and roasted sweet potato

Lunch: Kale salad with roasted carrots, chickpeas, dried cranberries, and light tahini dressing

Dinner: Baked sweet potato topped with black bean and corn salsa, with sautéed spinach

Option 6

Breakfast: ¾ cup Greek yogurt with 1 tablespoon peanut butter and 1 teaspoon dark chocolate chips

Lunch: Warm quinoa bowl with kale, roasted Brussels sprouts, raw sunflower seeds, and light lemon-tahini sauce

Dinner: Spaghetti squash with mushroom and lentil marinara

Even Days

Choose any of the following options to substitute into the main program for even days only.

Option 1

Breakfast: ¾ cup Greek yogurt with 1 tablespoon chia seeds and blueberries

Lunch: Roasted beet and goat cheese salad with arugula and walnuts (or try the Roasted Beet and Goat Cheese Salad recipe on page 233)

Snack: 10 to 12 raw almonds

Dinner: Baked chicken breast (4 ounces) with roasted Brussels sprouts and butternut squash

Option 2

Breakfast: Apple slices with 2 tablespoons almond butter

Lunch: Buckwheat soba noodles with tofu, edamame, carrots, and light miso-ginger dressing

Snack: 1 hard-boiled egg

Dinner: Grilled shrimp (4 ounces) with roasted asparagus and ½ cup brown rice

Option 3

Breakfast: ¾ cup Greek yogurt with chopped dried apricots

Lunch: Warm Quinoa and Roasted Vegetable Bowl (page 232) with zucchini, cherry tomatoes, and bell peppers

Snack: 1 orange

Dinner: Grilled mackerel (4 ounces) with roasted carrots and turnips, and steamed broccoli

Option 4

Breakfast: Slice of whole-grain toast with 2 scrambled eggs and spinach

Lunch: Roasted vegetable salad with arugula, sweet potatoes, red onion, and balsamic glaze (or try the Mediterranean Chickpea Salad on page 220)

Snack: ¼ cup raw pecans

Dinner: Baked chicken thigh (4 ounces) with roasted Brussels sprouts and mashed cauliflower

Option 5

Breakfast: Oatmeal with 1 tablespoon almond butter and strawberries

Lunch: Brown rice and edamame salad with shredded red cabbage, carrots, and light ginger-sesame dressing

Snack: 1 ounce mixed nuts

Dinner: Baked haddock (4 ounces) with roasted butternut squash and steamed green beans

Option 6

Breakfast: ½ cup low-fat cottage cheese with diced mango

Lunch: Farro salad with roasted mushrooms, kale, and light balsamic vinaigrette dressing

Snack: Carrot sticks with 2 tablespoons hummus

Dinner: Grilled turkey breast (4 ounces) with sweet potato fries and sautéed spinach

WEEK 3

Day 1

Breakfast: Veggie omelet with 2 eggs, peppers, onions, and mushrooms

Lunch: Arugula salad with roasted Brussels sprouts, pomegranate seeds, and balsamic glaze

Dinner: Baked sweet potato stuffed with black beans, corn, avocado, and salsa (or try the Stuffed Acorn Squash recipe on page 240)

Day 2

Breakfast: ½ cup chia pudding with raspberries

Lunch: Quinoa salad with mixed greens, cucumber, olives, and light lemon–olive oil dressing

Dinner: Spaghetti squash with marinara sauce and sautéed mushrooms (or try the Lentil Bolognese with Whole Wheat Spaghetti recipe on page 219)

Day 3

Breakfast: Protein waffle with ½ cup Greek yogurt and mixed berries

Lunch: Roasted beet salad with goat cheese, walnuts, and mixed greens (or try the Beet and Quinoa Salad recipe on page 199)

Dinner: Stir-fry with lentils, carrots, kale, and miso-tahini sauce

Day 4

Breakfast: Slice of whole-grain toast topped with ½ mashed avocado (or try the Avocado Toast with Tomato and Egg recipe on page 188)

Lunch: Chickpea salad with diced bell peppers, parsley, cucumbers, and light lemon-tahini dressing

Dinner: Baked acorn squash filled with wild rice, dried cranberries, and a few chopped nuts

Day 5

Breakfast: Breakfast burrito with 2 scrambled eggs, black beans, and salsa in a whole-grain tortilla

Lunch: Mixed greens salad with edamame, avocado, and light sesame dressing

Dinner: Vegetable curry with cauliflower, zucchini, and coconut milk over ½ cup quinoa (or try the Coconut Curry Vegetable Stew recipe on page 206)

Day 6

Breakfast: Breakfast bowl with ½ cup cooked brown rice, 1 scrambled egg, and ½ avocado, sliced

Lunch: Roasted vegetable salad with sweet potatoes, Brussels sprouts, kale, and light vinaigrette dressing (or try the Roasted Beet and Goat Cheese Salad recipe on page 233)

Dinner: Baked zucchini boats stuffed with quinoa, black beans, and light tomato sauce

Day 7

Breakfast: Egg white scramble with 1 cup liquid egg whites and 1 small turkey sausage

Lunch: Arugula and spinach salad with roasted red peppers, artichokes, and balsamic drizzle

Dinner: Stir-fry with tofu (6 ounces), bok choy, mushrooms, and ginger-soy sauce

Alternate Options
All Days

Choose any of the following options to substitute into the main program for any day you want.

Option 1

Breakfast: ¾ cup low-fat cottage cheese with ¼ cup sliced raw almonds and peaches

Lunch: Roasted cauliflower and chickpea salad with arugula, pomegranate seeds, and light balsamic dressing

Dinner: Baked tofu (6 ounces) with steamed broccoli and garlic-ginger sauce

Option 2

Breakfast: Oatmeal with 1 tablespoon chia seeds and blueberries

Lunch: Farro salad with mixed greens, roasted beets, edamame, and light tahini dressing

Dinner: Baked bell peppers stuffed with quinoa, kale, and feta cheese

Option 3

Breakfast: Egg scramble with 2 eggs and sautéed spinach and slice of whole-grain toast

Lunch: Spinach and avocado salad with roasted chickpeas, pumpkin seeds, and light lemon–olive oil dressing

Dinner: Lentil stew with carrots, celery, and tomatoes, with steamed green beans

Option 4

Breakfast: ¾ cup Greek yogurt with 2 tablespoons low-sugar granola and strawberries

Lunch: Arugula and roasted vegetable salad with sweet potatoes, red onion, and balsamic glaze

Dinner: Stir-fry with tempeh (6 ounces), snap peas, bell peppers, and ginger-soy sauce

Option 5

Breakfast: Smoothie (12 ounces) with 1 cup almond milk, 25 grams protein powder, ½ banana, 1 tablespoon peanut butter, and 1 cup spinach

Lunch: Roasted chickpea and carrot salad with kale, dried cranberries, and light lemon-tahini dressing

Dinner: Baked acorn squash filled with wild rice and mushrooms

Option 6

Breakfast: 1 cup low-fat cottage cheese with 1 tablespoon almond slices and ½ cup pineapple chunks

Lunch: Lentil and roasted vegetable salad with arugula, pomegranate seeds, and light vinaigrette dressing

Dinner: Baked acorn squash filled with black beans and corn with chili powder (or try the Zucchini Noodles with Pesto and Cherry Tomatoes recipe on page 248)

WEEK 4

Day 1

Breakfast: Slice of whole-grain toast topped with ¼ mashed avocado and 1 sliced hard-boiled egg

Lunch: Lentil and quinoa bowl with chopped spinach, red onion, and light olive oil dressing

Snack: Cherry tomatoes with 1 ounce mozzarella cheese

Dinner: Baked tilapia (6 ounces) with lemon, garlic, steamed asparagus, and mashed cauliflower (or try the Grilled Mahi-Mahi with Mango Salsa recipe on page 211)

Day 2

Breakfast: Egg scramble with 2 egg whites, 1 whole egg, mushrooms, bell peppers, and 1 teaspoon olive oil (or try the Greek Yogurt Parfait recipe on page 191)

Lunch: Hummus and veggie wrap with mixed veggies and avocado in a whole-grain tortilla

Snack: 1 orange

Dinner: Grilled flank steak (4 ounces) with roasted Brussels sprouts and baked sweet potato

Day 3

Breakfast: Whole-grain English muffin with 1 tablespoon almond butter and sliced banana

Lunch: Kale and chickpea salad with light tahini dressing (or try the Mediterranean Chickpea Salad recipe on page 220)

Snack: Celery sticks with 1 tablespoon almond butter

Dinner: Baked chicken breast (4 ounces) with roasted zucchini and ½ cup quinoa (or try the Dijon-Panko Chicken Tray Bake with Roasted Vegetables recipe on page 209)

Day 4

Breakfast: 1 cup cooked quinoa with almond milk, diced apple, and cinnamon

Lunch: Spaghetti squash with marinara sauce and grilled mushrooms

Snack: 1 apple

Dinner: Baked salmon (4 ounces) with sautéed spinach and roasted carrots (or try the Lemon-Garlic Baked Salmon recipe on page 215)

Day 5

Breakfast: Small whole wheat tortilla with 2 scrambled eggs and 2 tablespoons salsa

Lunch: Black bean and corn salad with mixed greens and light lime dressing

Snack: 10 to 12 raw almonds

Dinner: Grilled shrimp (4 ounces) with quinoa and roasted cauliflower (or try the Thai Red Curry with Shrimp recipe on page 242)

Day 6

Breakfast: 2 hard-boiled eggs, 10 to 12 raw almonds, and 1 orange

Lunch: Mediterranean grain bowl with farro, chickpeas, cucumber, cherry tomatoes, and feta cheese

Snack: Carrot sticks with 2 tablespoons hummus

Dinner: Grilled tofu (6 ounces) with roasted sweet potatoes and steamed broccoli

Day 7

Breakfast: Slice of whole-grain toast topped with 2 tablespoons mashed low-fat cottage cheese and ¼ sliced avocado

Lunch: Spinach salad with walnuts, dried cranberries, goat cheese, and light balsamic vinaigrette dressing

Snack: 1 hard-boiled egg

Dinner: Baked cod (4 ounces) with roasted Brussels sprouts and ½ cup wild rice (or try the Mediterranean Cod with Tomatoes and Olives recipe on page 221)

Alternate Options

All Days

Choose any of the following options to substitute into the main program for any day you want.

Option 1

Breakfast: 1 cup high-fiber, low-sugar cereal with low-fat milk and strawberries

Lunch: Barley and roasted beet salad with goat cheese and arugula

Snack: 1 hard-boiled egg

Dinner: Grilled shrimp (4 ounces) with roasted cauliflower and wild rice

Option 2

Breakfast: Oatmeal with 1 tablespoon peanut butter and 1 teaspoon honey

Lunch: Lentil and roasted carrot salad with mixed greens and light lemon-tahini dressing

Snack: ½ cup edamame

Dinner: Baked trout (4 ounces) with roasted Brussels sprouts and mashed sweet potatoes

Option 3

Breakfast: Banana with 2 tablespoons peanut butter

Lunch: Chickpea and avocado salad with cherry tomatoes, cucumber, and light olive oil dressing

Snack: Celery sticks with 1 tablespoon sunflower seed butter

Dinner: Grilled pork tenderloin (4 ounces) with sautéed kale and roasted parsnips

Option 4

Breakfast: ½ cup Greek yogurt with pomegranate seeds

Lunch: Quinoa salad with roasted bell peppers, spinach, chickpeas, and light lemon vinaigrette dressing

Snack: ¼ cup raw walnuts

Dinner: Baked cod (4 ounces) with steamed asparagus and brown rice

Option 5

Breakfast: Breakfast bowl with ½ cup brown rice, 1 scrambled egg, and ½ sliced avocado

Lunch: Warm barley and mixed vegetable bowl with sautéed mushrooms, zucchini, and arugula

Snack: ¼ cup pumpkin seeds

Dinner: Grilled lamb chop (4 ounces) with roasted carrots and baked sweet potato

Option 6

Breakfast: ¾ cup Greek yogurt with 1 tablespoon pumpkin seeds and blackberries

Lunch: Roasted chickpea and kale salad with light tahini dressing

Snack: 1 pear

Dinner: Grilled bison steak (4 ounces) with mashed cauliflower and roasted Brussels sprouts

WEEK 5

Day 1

Breakfast: Small whole-grain tortilla with 3 egg whites and 2 tablespoons shredded cheese

Lunch: Spinach salad with roasted chickpeas, shredded carrots, raw sunflower seeds, and light lemon–olive oil dressing (or try the Quinoa and Roasted Vegetable Bowl recipe on page 232)

Dinner: Baked falafel with cucumber-tomato salad and a dollop of hummus

Day 2

Breakfast: Oatmeal with 1 tablespoon almond butter and ½ tablespoon chia seeds

Lunch: Grilled vegetable and hummus wrap with grilled zucchini, bell peppers, and onion in a whole-grain tortilla

Snack: 1 small apple

Dinner: Baked chicken breast (4 ounces) with sautéed kale and ½ cup quinoa (or try the Lemon-Herb Grilled Chicken recipe on page 217)

Day 3

Breakfast: Whole-grain English muffin with 1 scrambled egg and tomato slice

Lunch: Arugula salad with roasted asparagus, artichokes, pine nuts, and light balsamic dressing

Dinner: Baked portobello mushroom cap stuffed with barley, spinach, and feta cheese

Day 4

Breakfast: ¾ cup low-fat cottage cheese with ¼ cup sliced raw almonds and blueberries

Lunch: Warm lentil salad with arugula, roasted cherry tomatoes, and light vinaigrette dressing (or try the Curried Cauliflower and Lentils recipe on page 207)

Snack: 1 orange

Dinner: Grilled salmon (4 ounces) with roasted sweet potatoes and steamed asparagus

Day 5

Breakfast: Egg scramble with 2 egg whites, 1 whole egg, feta cheese, and spinach (or try the Sweet Potato and Kale Frittata recipe on page 194)

Lunch: Brown rice and black bean salad with corn, red onion, cilantro, and light lime dressing

Dinner: Sweet potato and kale hash with nutritional yeast

Day 6

Breakfast: Baked sweet potato and 1 scrambled egg

Lunch: Mixed bean chili with black beans, kidney beans, and diced tomatoes (or try the Deviled Eggs recipe on page 208)

Snack: ¼ cup raw walnuts

Dinner: Stir-fry with shrimp (6 medium), bell peppers, broccoli, and cauliflower rice

Day 7

Breakfast: 1 cup kefir with 1 tablespoon chia seeds and blueberries

Lunch: Warm quinoa bowl with roasted cauliflower, chickpeas, and lemon-tahini sauce (or try the Chicken and Quinoa Bowl recipe on page 202)

Dinner: Eggplant caponata with steamed green beans

Alternate Options
Odd Days

Choose any of the following options to substitute into the main program for odd days only.

Option 1

Breakfast: 2 hard-boiled eggs, 10 to 12 raw almonds, and 1 orange

Lunch: Quinoa salad with mixed greens, artichoke hearts, roasted red peppers, and pine nuts

Dinner: Baked portobello mushroom cap stuffed with lentils, spinach, and sun-dried tomatoes

Option 2

Breakfast: 2 banana protein pancakes with light syrup

Lunch: Spinach salad with roasted red peppers, pine nuts, and light lemon-tahini dressing

Dinner: Baked sweet potato stuffed with kale, chickpeas, and light tahini drizzle

Option 3

Breakfast: Banana with 2 tablespoons almond butter

Lunch: Quinoa and avocado bowl with mixed greens, roasted butternut squash, and light balsamic glaze

Dinner: Stir-fry with tofu (6 ounces), snap peas, mushrooms, and garlic-ginger sauce

Option 4

Breakfast: ¾ cup Greek yogurt with mixed berries

Lunch: Farro salad with arugula, roasted carrots, walnuts, and pomegranate seeds

Dinner: Baked bell peppers stuffed with brown rice, black beans, corn, and salsa

Option 5

Breakfast: ½ cup Greek yogurt with ¼ cup raw pecans and sliced banana

Lunch: Kale salad with roasted beets, chickpeas, and light lemon-tahini dressing

Dinner: Spaghetti squash with tomato and lentil marinara, topped with fresh basil

Option 6

Breakfast: 1 cup diced honeydew melon with ½ cup low-fat cottage cheese

Lunch: Spinach and quinoa salad with roasted asparagus, raw sunflower seeds, and light lemon–olive oil dressing

Dinner: Baked acorn squash filled with wild rice, dried cranberries, and walnuts

Even Days

Choose any of the following options to substitute into the main program for even days only.

Option 1

Breakfast: ½ cup Greek yogurt with mixed berries

Lunch: Warm lentil and spinach salad with roasted pumpkin and balsamic glaze

Snack: 1 hard-boiled egg

Dinner: Grilled salmon (4 ounces) with roasted parsnips and steamed broccoli

Option 2

Breakfast: Protein shake or smoothie (12 ounces) 200 calories or less

Lunch: Spinach salad with pomegranate seeds, walnuts, avocado, and light balsamic vinaigrette dressing (or try the Quinoa and Black Bean Salad on page 231)

Snack: ½ cup edamame

Dinner: Baked chicken thigh (4 ounces) with roasted cauliflower and sautéed zucchini

Option 3

Breakfast: Apple slices with 1 tablespoon almond butter

Lunch: Spicy roasted chickpea and kale bowl with tahini dressing

Snack: Cucumber slices with 2 tablespoons hummus

Dinner: Grilled swordfish (4 ounces) with roasted butternut squash and sautéed kale

Option 4

Breakfast: ½ cup Greek yogurt with chopped dates and honey drizzle

Lunch: Chickpea and bulgur salad with fresh mint, parsley, cucumber, and light lemon–olive oil dressing

Snack: 1 apple

Dinner: Grilled scallops (4 ounces) with roasted baby carrots and steamed Swiss chard

Option 5

Breakfast: Banana with 1 tablespoon almond butter

Lunch: Lentil and roasted beet salad with arugula and goat cheese

Snack: 10 to 12 raw almonds

Dinner: Baked trout (4 ounces) with mashed sweet potatoes and sautéed green beans

Option 6

Breakfast: 1 cup mixed fruit with ¼ cup Greek yogurt
Lunch: Black bean, corn, and avocado salad with red onion and light lime dressing
Snack: ½ cup low-fat cottage cheese with mixed berries
Dinner: Grilled chicken breast (4 ounces) with roasted zucchini and wild rice

WEEK 6

Day 1

Breakfast: Small whole wheat pita with 3 tablespoons hummus, 2 sliced hard-boiled eggs, and cucumber slices

Lunch: Farro salad with arugula, roasted red peppers, olives, and light lemon-tahini dressing

Dinner: 3 cabbage rolls, approximately 3–4 inches long, stuffed with lentils, carrots, and brown rice (or try the Spinach and Feta Stuffed Peppers recipe on page 238)

Day 2

Breakfast: ¾ cup plain kefir with ½ cup pineapple chunks, 2 tablespoons oats, and 1 tablespoon hemp seeds

Lunch: Chickpea and quinoa salad with chopped spinach, red onion, and light tahini dressing (or try the Caprese Salad with Avocado recipe on page 200)

Snack: 1 pear

Dinner: Baked tilapia (4 ounces) with roasted Brussels sprouts and mashed cauliflower

Day 3

Breakfast: Breakfast burrito with corn tortilla, 1 scrambled egg, black beans, salsa, and 1 tablespoon queso fresco

Lunch: Spinach salad with pomegranate seeds, walnuts, avocado, and light balsamic vinaigrette dressing

Dinner: Stir-fry with tempeh (6 ounces), broccoli, bell peppers, and garlic-ginger sauce (or try the Grilled Vegetable Skewers recipe on page 212)

Day 4

Breakfast: ½ cup cooked barley with ½ cup diced pear, 1 tablespoon raw pecans, and cinnamon

Lunch: Spinach salad with strawberries, raw almonds, goat cheese, and light balsamic vinaigrette dressing

Snack: 10 to 12 mixed nuts

Dinner: Grilled tofu (4 ounces) with roasted carrots and sautéed kale (or try the Spinach and Mushroom Quesadilla recipe on page 239)

Day 5

Breakfast: Smoothie (12 ounces) with 1 cup unsweetened soy milk, 25 grams protein powder, ½ cup frozen cherries, and 1 tablespoon almond butter (or try the Chia Seed Pudding with Berries recipe on page 190)

Lunch: Mixed greens with roasted carrots, quinoa, chickpeas, and light turmeric-ginger dressing

Dinner: Baked sweet potato with black beans, corn, and light salsa (or try the Zucchini Noodles with Pesto and Cherry Tomatoes on page 248)

Day 6

Breakfast: ¾ cup Greek yogurt with 1 tablespoon walnuts, grated carrot, and raisins

Lunch: Bulgur wheat salad with chickpeas, parsley, red onion, cucumber, and light lemon–olive oil dressing

Snack: 1 orange

Dinner: Baked chicken thigh (4 ounces) with steamed green beans and ½ cup wild rice (or try the Baked Chicken with Vegetables recipe on page 197)

Day 7

Breakfast: ½ cup low-fat cottage cheese with diced cucumber, cherry tomatoes, and light olive oil drizzle

Lunch: Roasted vegetable bowl with sweet potatoes, Brussels sprouts, kale, and tahini sauce (or try the Spicy Shrimp and Quinoa Bowl recipe on page 236)

Dinner: Butternut squash soup with mixed greens

Alternate Options

Odd Days

Choose any of the following options to substitute into the main program for odd days only.

Option 1

Breakfast: Protein shake (12 ounces) with 1 cup unsweetened almond milk, ½ cup pumpkin puree, 25 grams vanilla protein powder, and pumpkin spice

Lunch: Mixed greens salad with roasted Brussels sprouts, pumpkin seeds, and light vinaigrette dressing

Dinner: Eggplant and zucchini stew with tomatoes, onions, and feta cheese

Option 2

Breakfast: 2 scrambled egg whites with baked plantain

Lunch: Tabbouleh with bulgur, parsley, diced cucumber, cherry tomatoes, and light lemon–olive oil dressing

Dinner: Cauliflower and chickpea curry served over ½ cup brown rice

Option 3

Breakfast: Rice cake with 2 tablespoons peanut butter and sliced strawberries

Lunch: Arugula salad with roasted red onion, chickpeas, avocado, and light balsamic dressing

Dinner: Baked or grilled salmon (6 ounces) with roasted sweet potatoes and sautéed spinach (or try the Zucchini Noodles with Pesto and Cherry Tomatoes recipe on page 248)

Option 4

Breakfast: Slice of whole-grain toast topped with mashed white beans, arugula, and paprika

Lunch: Quinoa salad with kale, roasted sweet potatoes, raw pecans, and light tahini dressing

Dinner: Baked portobello mushroom cap stuffed with lentils, spinach, and sun-dried tomatoes

Option 5

Breakfast: Roasted breakfast potatoes (5 ounces) with 1 poached egg and salsa verde

Lunch: Roasted vegetable bowl with Brussels sprouts, carrots, chickpeas, and light lemon–olive oil dressing

Dinner: Stir-fry with tempeh (6 ounces), bok choy, snap peas, and ginger-tamari sauce

Option 6

Breakfast: 1 cup unsweetened soy yogurt with 2 tablespoons low-sugar granola and blackberries

Lunch: Spinach salad with roasted butternut squash, dried cranberries, walnuts, and light maple-balsamic dressing

Dinner: Baked bell peppers stuffed with black beans, vegetables, and shredded cheese

Even Days

Choose any of the following options to substitute into the main program for even days only.

Option 1

Breakfast: Oatmeal with 1 tablespoon tahini, 1 teaspoon maple syrup, and sliced banana

Lunch: Mediterranean quinoa bowl with chickpeas, olives, sun-dried tomatoes, and feta cheese

Snack: 1 hard-boiled egg

Dinner: Baked swordfish (4 ounces) with roasted Brussels sprouts and baked sweet potato

Option 2

Breakfast: ¾ cup Greek yogurt with pomegranate seeds

Lunch: Kale and roasted vegetable salad with light tahini dressing

Snack: 1 apple

Dinner: Grilled pork tenderloin (4 ounces) with sautéed spinach and roasted parsnips

Option 3

Breakfast: Banana with 1 tablespoon almond butter

Lunch: Warm barley salad with roasted butternut squash, arugula, and light balsamic glaze

Snack: Carrot sticks with 2 tablespoons hummus

Dinner: Baked cod (4 ounces) with steamed asparagus and quinoa

Option 4

Breakfast: ¾ cup low-fat cottage cheese with ½ cup diced mango

Lunch: Spinach and farro salad with walnuts, dried cranberries, and goat cheese

Snack: 1 pear

Dinner: Grilled shrimp (4 ounces) with roasted cauliflower and mashed sweet potatoes

Option 5

Breakfast: Protein shake (12 ounces) with 1 cup low-fat milk, ½ cup diced papaya, 25 grams protein powder, and 1 tablespoon ground flaxseed

Lunch: Mixed greens salad with roasted chickpeas, cucumber, cherry tomatoes, and light lemon–olive oil dressing

Snack: 10 to 12 raw cashews

Dinner: Baked chicken thigh (4 ounces) with sautéed kale and roasted carrots

Option 6

Breakfast: Slice of whole-grain toast topped with 1 tablespoon peanut butter, 1 tablespoon crushed peanuts, and apple slices

Lunch: Roasted eggplant and chickpea bowl with quinoa and tahini drizzle

Snack: Cucumber slices with 2 tablespoons tzatziki

Dinner: Grilled lamb chop (4 ounces) with roasted Brussels sprouts and mashed parsnips

WEEK 7

Day 1

Breakfast: 2 scrambled eggs with sautéed spinach and slice of whole-grain toast

Lunch: Kale salad with edamame, bell peppers, sesame seeds, and light miso-ginger dressing (or try the Tuna Salad with Avocado and Chickpeas recipe on page 245)

Dinner: Black bean and vegetable chili with shredded cheese

Day 2

Breakfast: 1 cup low-fat cottage cheese with 1 tablespoon almond slices and pineapple chunks

Lunch: Tabbouleh with parsley, bulgur, tomatoes, cucumber, and light lemon–olive oil dressing

Dinner: Baked acorn squash filled with quinoa and dried cranberries

Day 3

Breakfast: Slice of whole-grain toast topped with ¼ mashed avocado and 1 sliced hard-boiled egg

Lunch: Lentil salad with diced tomatoes, red onion, cilantro, and light cumin-lime dressing

Dinner: Chickpea and spinach curry over cauliflower rice

Day 4

Breakfast: Whole-grain English muffin with 1 tablespoon almond butter and sliced banana

Lunch: Mixed greens with roasted beets, feta cheese, pumpkin seeds, and balsamic glaze

Dinner: Stir-fry with tofu (6 ounces), bok choy, snap peas, and tamari sauce (or try the Oysters and Mignonette recipe on page 225)

Day 5

Breakfast: Small whole wheat tortilla with 2 scrambled eggs and salsa

Lunch: Arugula salad with roasted butternut squash, pomegranate seeds, and walnuts

Dinner: Baked bell peppers stuffed with brown rice, black beans, and corn

Day 6

Breakfast: ½ cup low-fat cottage cheese with raspberries (or try the Overnight Oats with Almonds and Apples recipe on page 192)

Lunch: Spinach salad with quinoa, roasted zucchini, pine nuts, and light lemon-tahini dressing

Dinner: Miso-glazed eggplant with steamed broccoli

Day 7

Breakfast: Oatmeal with 1 tablespoon walnuts and diced pear

Lunch: Warm quinoa bowl with broccoli, red onion, and tahini sauce

Dinner: Spaghetti squash with lentil-tomato ragù and fresh basil (or try the Aglio e Olio recipe on page 196)

Alternate Options
All Days

Choose any of the following options to substitute into the main program for any day you want.

The New Menopause Kitchen Meal Plan

Option 1

Breakfast: Smoothie (12 ounces) with 1 cup coconut water, 25 grams protein powder, and 1 cup frozen mango

Lunch: Lentil and arugula salad with roasted carrots, pumpkin seeds, and light lemon-tahini dressing

Dinner: Baked sweet potato with black beans, corn, and light salsa

Option 2

Breakfast: Slice of whole-grain toast topped with 2 tablespoons mashed low-fat cottage cheese and ¼ sliced avocado

Lunch: Quinoa salad with roasted cauliflower, kale, and pomegranate seeds

Dinner: Eggplant caponata with steamed green beans

Option 3

Breakfast: Oatmeal with 1 tablespoon peanut butter and 1 teaspoon honey

Lunch: Arugula salad with roasted red peppers, olives, artichokes, and balsamic glaze

Dinner: Stir-fry with tofu (6 ounces), bell peppers, mushrooms, and garlic-ginger sauce

Option 4

Breakfast: ¾ cup Greek yogurt with 1 tablespoon pumpkin seeds and blackberries

Lunch: Spinach salad with avocado, roasted chickpeas, and light lemon–olive oil dressing

Dinner: Baked acorn squash filled with barley and mixed vegetables

Option 5

Breakfast: Breakfast bowl with ½ cup cooked brown rice, 1 scrambled egg, and ½ sliced avocado

Lunch: Arugula salad with roasted eggplant, pine nuts, and light lemon–olive oil dressing

Dinner: Baked sweet potato topped with sautéed kale, chickpeas, and tahini drizzle

Option 6

Breakfast: Breakfast burrito with whole-grain tortilla, 3 scrambled egg whites, and 2 tablespoons shredded cheese

Lunch: Mixed greens salad with roasted carrots, pumpkin seeds, and light ginger dressing

Dinner: Cauliflower steak with roasted Brussels sprouts and turmeric dressing

WEEK 8

Day 1

Breakfast: ¾ cup Greek yogurt with mixed berries

Lunch: Lentil and vegetable soup with slice of whole-grain bread

Snack: Carrot sticks with 2 tablespoons hummus

Dinner: Grilled turkey burger (6 ounces, no bun) with roasted Brussels sprouts and baked sweet potato

Day 2

Breakfast: 2 hard-boiled eggs and slice of whole-grain toast

Lunch: Kale and avocado salad with quinoa, chickpeas, and light lemon-tahini dressing

Snack: 10 to 12 raw almonds

Dinner: Baked cod (4 ounces) with roasted butternut squash and steamed broccoli

Day 3

Breakfast: ½ cup low-fat cottage cheese with raspberries

Lunch: Mediterranean grain bowl with farro, cucumber, cherry tomatoes, olives, and feta cheese

Snack: 1 hard-boiled egg

Dinner: Grilled shrimp (4 ounces) with roasted sweet potatoes and sautéed spinach (or try the Lemon-Garlic Shrimp with Quinoa recipe on page 216)

Day 4

Breakfast: Oatmeal with 1 tablespoon almond butter and ½ tablespoon chia seeds

Lunch: Black bean and corn salad with avocado, red onion, and light lime dressing

Snack: Celery sticks with 1 tablespoon almond butter

Dinner: Grilled chicken breast (4 ounces) with roasted zucchini and ½ cup brown rice (or try the Chicken in Salsa Verde recipe on page 203)

Day 5

Breakfast: Banana with 2 tablespoons peanut butter

Lunch: Quinoa and chickpea salad with arugula, red bell pepper, and light olive oil dressing

Snack: Cucumber slices with 2 tablespoons tzatziki

Dinner: Baked salmon (4 ounces) with roasted carrots and steamed kale

Day 6

Breakfast: Whole-grain English muffin with 1 scrambled egg and tomato slice

Lunch: Mixed bean salad with bell peppers, red onion, parsley, and light vinaigrette dressing

Snack: ¼ cup raw walnuts

Dinner: Grilled tofu (4 ounces) with roasted Brussels sprouts and mashed sweet potato (or try the Mystic, Connecticut–Style Portuguese Stew recipe on page 224)

Day 7

Breakfast: ¾ cup low-fat cottage cheese with ¼ cup sliced raw almonds and blueberries

Lunch: Hummus and vegetable wrap with mixed greens, cucumber, and bell peppers in a whole-grain tortilla

Snack: 1 hard-boiled egg

Dinner: Baked tilapia (4 ounces) with steamed asparagus and ½ cup wild rice (or try the Whole Wheat Pasta with Spinach and Chickpeas recipe on page 247)

Alternate Options
All Days

Choose any of the following options to substitute into the main program for any day you want.

Option 1

Breakfast: Apple slices with 2 tablespoons sunflower seed butter

Lunch: Freekeh salad with roasted red pepper, cucumber, and feta cheese

Snack: ½ cup edamame

Dinner: Grilled salmon (4 ounces) with steamed green beans and brown rice

Option 2

Breakfast: Slice of whole-grain toast topped with 1 tablespoon peanut butter and raspberries

Lunch: Quinoa and roasted vegetable salad with chopped kale, carrots, and light vinaigrette dressing

Snack: Celery sticks with 1 tablespoon almond butter

Dinner: Baked halibut (4 ounces) with roasted sweet potatoes and sautéed spinach

Option 3

Breakfast: ½ cup low-fat cottage cheese with mixed berries

Lunch: Bulgur salad with chickpeas, cucumber, mint, and light lemon–olive oil dressing

Snack: 1 hard-boiled egg

Dinner: Grilled turkey breast (4 ounces) with roasted broccoli and wild rice

Option 4

Breakfast: ½ cup Greek yogurt with ½ cup pineapple chunks and 1 tablespoon chia seeds

Lunch: Lentil and kale soup with slice of whole-grain bread

Snack: ¼ cup raw walnuts

Dinner: Baked trout (4 ounces) with mashed cauliflower and roasted Brussels sprouts

Option 5

Breakfast: Egg scramble with 2 egg whites, 1 whole egg, feta cheese, and spinach

Lunch: Warm quinoa and black bean bowl with avocado, red onion, and light lime dressing

Snack: Carrot sticks with 2 tablespoons hummus

Dinner: Grilled scallops (4 ounces) with roasted baby carrots and sautéed kale

Option 6

Breakfast: Baked sweet potato and 1 scrambled egg

Lunch: Roasted fennel and citrus salad with mixed greens, olives, and light vinaigrette dressing

Snack: ½ cup low-fat cottage cheese with kiwi

Dinner: Baked monkfish (4 ounces) with steamed green beans and roasted fingerling potatoes

WEEK 9

Day 1

Breakfast: 2 banana protein pancakes with light syrup

Lunch: Mixed greens with roasted chickpeas, avocado, shredded carrots, and light lemon–olive oil dressing

Dinner: Coconut milk–based vegetable curry with eggplant, bell peppers, and brown rice

Day 2

Breakfast: ¾ cup Greek yogurt with 1 tablespoon chia seeds

Lunch: Spinach and feta salad with walnuts, dried cranberries, and light balsamic vinaigrette dressing

Snack: 1 orange

Dinner: Grilled chicken thigh (4 ounces) with roasted Brussels sprouts and mashed cauliflower (or try the Portuguese Chicken recipe on page 229)

Day 3

Breakfast: Breakfast bowl with ½ cup brown rice, 1 scrambled egg, and ½ sliced avocado

Lunch: Barley salad with roasted beets, arugula, goat cheese, and light balsamic vinaigrette dressing

Dinner: 1 baked zucchini boat stuffed with quinoa, lentils, tomatoes, and feta cheese (or try the Gumbo Z'herbes recipe on page 213)

Day 4

Breakfast: Small whole wheat pita with 3 tablespoons hummus, 2 sliced hard-boiled eggs, and cucumber slices

Lunch: Roasted chickpea and kale salad with avocado, red onion, and light lemon–olive oil dressing (or try the Tomato Basil Soup recipe on page 244)

Snack: ½ cup edamame

Dinner: Grilled swordfish (4 ounces) with roasted red potatoes and steamed green beans

Day 5

Breakfast: 2 scrambled eggs, 2 slices turkey bacon, and ½ cup diced melon

Lunch: Spinach salad with roasted Brussels sprouts, raw almonds, dried cranberries, and light lemon–olive oil dressing

Dinner: Stir-fry with tempeh (6 ounces), mushrooms, bok choy, and sesame-ginger sauce (or try the Vegetable Stir-Fry with Tofu recipe on page 246)

Day 6

Breakfast: ½ cup low-fat cottage cheese with ½ cup sliced peaches

Lunch: Buckwheat soba noodle salad with shredded cabbage, carrots, bell peppers, and light sesame dressing

Snack: 1 pear

Dinner: Baked halibut (4 ounces) with sautéed Swiss chard and roasted beets

Day 7

Breakfast: ¾ cup Greek yogurt with ¼ cup low-sugar granola and blueberries

Lunch: Arugula salad with roasted carrots, pumpkin seeds, pomegranate seeds, and light tahini dressing

Dinner: Cauliflower and chickpea stew with turmeric, ginger, and coconut milk (or try the Pasta Primavera with Whole Wheat Penne recipe on page 228)

Alternate Options
Odd Days

Choose any of the following options to substitute into the main program for odd days only.

Option 1

Breakfast: Breakfast burrito with low-carb tortilla, 2 scrambled egg whites, and 2 tablespoons shredded cheese

Lunch: Warm quinoa bowl with arugula, roasted butternut squash, and dried cranberries

Dinner: Baked bell peppers stuffed with lentils, quinoa, and feta cheese

Option 2

Breakfast: ½ cup low-fat cottage cheese with 1 cup diced mango and 1 tablespoon chia seeds

Lunch: Tabbouleh with parsley, bulgur, tomatoes, and light lemon-mint dressing

Dinner: Roasted spaghetti squash with garlic-mushroom sauce

Option 3

Breakfast: 2 hard-boiled eggs and slice of whole-grain toast

Lunch: Farro salad with spinach, roasted sweet potatoes, and pomegranate seeds

Dinner: Eggplant stew with tomatoes, lentils, and sautéed spinach

Option 4

Breakfast: ½ cup ricotta cheese with 1 teaspoon honey and sliced strawberries

Lunch: Arugula and chickpea salad with roasted red onion and light balsamic vinaigrette dressing

Dinner: Baked acorn squash filled with black beans and corn

Option 5

Breakfast: Oatmeal with 1 tablespoon almond butter and 1 tablespoon chia seeds

Lunch: Spinach salad with roasted beets, walnuts, and goat cheese

Dinner: Zucchini fritters with mixed greens

Option 6

Breakfast: Whole-grain English muffin with 1 scrambled egg and tomato slice

Lunch: Mixed greens with avocado, roasted cauliflower, and light lemon-tahini dressing

Dinner: Stir-fry with tofu (6 ounces), snap peas, bell peppers, and sesame-ginger sauce

Even Days

Choose any of the following options to substitute into the main program for even days only.

Option 1

Breakfast: ½ cup Greek yogurt with raw sunflower seeds

Lunch: Warm spelt salad with roasted mushrooms, leeks, and light balsamic dressing

Snack: 15 pistachios

Dinner: Grilled chicken sausage (4 ounces) with roasted acorn squash and steamed broccoli

Option 2

Breakfast: Banana with 2 tablespoons cashew butter

Lunch: Kale and pomegranate salad with goat cheese, walnuts, and light lemon–olive oil dressing

Snack: 1 orange

Dinner: Baked pollock (4 ounces) with mashed parsnips and sautéed Swiss chard

Option 3

Breakfast: ½ cup low-fat cottage cheese with strawberries

Lunch: Chickpea and roasted red pepper wrap with spinach and tahini sauce in a whole-grain tortilla

Snack: 1 hard-boiled egg

Dinner: Grilled tuna steak (4 ounces) with roasted Brussels sprouts and quinoa

Option 4

Breakfast: Slice of whole-grain toast topped with 1 tablespoon peanut butter and raspberries

Lunch: Warm roasted cauliflower and lentil salad with light lemon-tahini dressing

Snack: 1 apple

Dinner: Baked chicken drumsticks (4 ounces) with roasted carrots and mashed sweet potatoes

Option 5

Breakfast: Egg scramble with 2 egg whites, 1 whole egg, feta cheese, and spinach

Lunch: Arugula and fennel salad with citrus segments and light vinaigrette dressing

Snack: ¼ cup pumpkin seeds

Dinner: Grilled bison burger (6 ounces, no bun) with roasted eggplant and steamed kale

Option 6

Breakfast: ½ cup Greek yogurt with 1 teaspoon ground flaxseed and mixed berries

Lunch: Spinach salad with roasted butternut squash, dried cranberries, and feta cheese

Snack: Cucumber slices with 2 tablespoons hummus

Dinner: Baked cod (4 ounces) with roasted beets and steamed asparagus

WEEK 10

Day 1

Breakfast: 2 scrambled egg whites with baked plantain (or try the Apple Cinnamon Oatmeal recipe on page 187)

Lunch: Spicy black bean and avocado wrap with spinach and salsa in a whole-grain tortilla

Dinner: Grilled pork tenderloin (4 ounces) with steamed broccoli and quinoa

Day 2

Breakfast: Oatmeal with 1 tablespoon tahini, 1 teaspoon maple syrup, and sliced banana

Lunch: Spinach and lentil salad with roasted pumpkin, feta cheese, and balsamic glaze

Snack: Celery sticks with 2 tablespoons guacamole

Dinner: Baked chicken thigh (4 ounces) with roasted parsnips and sautéed zucchini (or try the Coconut Curry Chicken recipe on page 205)

Day 3

Breakfast: 1 cup unsweetened soy yogurt with 2 tablespoons low-sugar granola and mixed berries

Lunch: Lentil and kale salad with roasted butternut squash and balsamic glaze (or try the Mediterranean Lentil Soup recipe on page 222)

Dinner: Baked eggplant rounds with tomato basil sauce and grated Parmesan cheese

Day 4

Breakfast: 2 scrambled eggs with sautéed spinach and slice of whole-grain toast (or try the Berry Oatmeal Bake recipe on page 189)

Lunch: Quinoa and avocado salad with diced cucumbers, cherry tomatoes, and light lime dressing

Snack: ½ cup Greek yogurt with ¼ cup raw pecans and berries

Dinner: Enchiladas with roasted sweet potato, black beans, and sautéed spinach (or try the Spinach and Feta Stuffed Chicken Breasts recipe on page 237)

Day 5

Breakfast: Smoothie (12 ounces) with 1 cup almond milk, 25 grams protein powder, ½ banana, ½ cup blueberries or strawberries, and 1 cup spinach

Lunch: Farro salad with sun-dried tomatoes, artichoke hearts, arugula, and light olive oil dressing

Dinner: Grilled scallops (4 ounces) with wild rice and steamed asparagus

Day 6

Breakfast: Slice of whole-grain toast topped with ¼ mashed avocado and 1 sliced hard-boiled egg

Lunch: Tabbouleh salad with bulgur, parsley, mint, tomato, and cucumber (or try the Pasta con le Sarde recipe on page 226)

Snack: 1 ounce raw cashews

Dinner: Baked trout (4 ounces) with roasted cauliflower and mashed sweet potatoes

Day 7

Breakfast: Breakfast burrito with small whole wheat tortilla, 2 scrambled eggs, and salsa (or try the Savory Oatmeal with Spinach and Eggs recipe on page 193)

Lunch: Roasted chickpea and vegetable bowl with broccoli, bell peppers, and turmeric-tahini sauce

Dinner: Zucchini noodles with marinara sauce, sautéed mushrooms, and pine nuts

Alternate Options
Odd Days

Choose any of the following options to substitute into the main program for odd days only.

Option 1

Breakfast: ½ cup Greek yogurt with blueberries

Lunch: Farro bowl with shredded cabbage, carrots, edamame, and light sesame-ginger dressing

Dinner: Grilled lamb skewers (4 ounces) with sautéed kale and roasted sweet potato wedges

Option 2

Breakfast: Breakfast bowl with ½ cup cooked brown rice, 1 scrambled egg, and ½ sliced avocado

Lunch: Bulgur salad with chopped tomatoes, parsley, cucumber, and light lemon–olive oil dressing

Dinner: Grilled turkey breast (4 ounces) with steamed cauliflower and mashed parsnips

Option 3

Breakfast: Apple slices with 1 tablespoon almond butter

Lunch: Warm barley and mixed vegetable bowl with roasted zucchini, bell peppers, and light olive oil drizzle

Dinner: Baked tilapia (4 ounces) with roasted Brussels sprouts and wild rice

Option 4

Breakfast: ½ cup Greek yogurt with pomegranate seeds

Lunch: Mixed greens salad with roasted chickpeas, olives, artichokes, and light lemon-tahini dressing

Dinner: Grilled shrimp (4 ounces) with roasted baby potatoes and sautéed spinach

Option 5

Breakfast: 1 cup mixed fruit with ¼ cup Greek yogurt

Lunch: Warm lentil salad with roasted eggplant, red onion, and light balsamic glaze

Dinner: Baked halibut (4 ounces) with roasted cauliflower and mashed sweet potatoes

Option 6

Breakfast: Apple slices with 2 tablespoons almond butter

Lunch: Roasted beet and carrot salad with arugula, walnuts, and light olive oil dressing

Dinner: Grilled turkey thigh (4 ounces) with sautéed kale and roasted squash

Even Days

Choose any of the following options to substitute into the main program for even days only.

Option 1

Breakfast: Apple slices with 1 tablespoon sunflower seed butter

Lunch: Roasted vegetable bowl with broccoli, carrots, chickpeas, and tahini drizzle

Snack: ½ cup low-fat cottage cheese with raspberries

Dinner: Butternut squash soup with arugula salad

Option 2

Breakfast: Baked sweet potato and 1 scrambled egg

Lunch: Quinoa and kale salad with edamame, bell peppers, and sesame seeds

Snack: Carrot sticks with 1 tablespoon tahini

Dinner: Baked portobello mushroom cap stuffed with lentils, with roasted zucchini

Option 3

Breakfast: ½ cup Greek yogurt with 1 cup sliced watermelon, banana, and strawberries

Lunch: Tabbouleh with quinoa, parsley, cucumbers, and light lemon–olive oil dressing

Snack: 1 cup mixed berries

Dinner: Baked tofu (6 ounces) with roasted Brussels sprouts

Option 4

Breakfast: ½ cup low-fat cottage cheese with ½ cup pineapple chunks

Lunch: Spinach salad with roasted chickpeas, pomegranate seeds, and light ginger dressing

Snack: Apple slices with 1 tablespoon peanut butter

Dinner: Baked zucchini boats stuffed with farro, lentils, and grated Parmesan cheese

Option 5

Breakfast: Slice of whole-grain toast topped with 1 tablespoon peanut butter and raspberries

Lunch: Farro and roasted vegetable salad with arugula, carrots, and light balsamic dressing

Snack: 10 to 12 raw almonds

Dinner: Cauliflower and chickpea curry with brown rice

Option 6

Breakfast: 1 cup Greek yogurt with mixed berries

Lunch: Arugula salad with roasted asparagus, pine nuts, and light lemon–olive oil dressing

Snack: Rice cake with 1 tablespoon almond butter

Dinner: Sweet potato and black bean chili with steamed kale

5

MENO-CISE: THE EXERCISE PLAN

The menopausal transition marks a profound shift not only in a woman's reproductive health but also in her overall physiology and metabolism. With the decline of estrogen—one of the body's most powerful regulatory hormones—women face a series of changes that can impact muscle mass, fat storage, bone density, metabolic rate, and even mood. Two of the most powerful tools a woman can embrace during this life phase are muscle building and weight management, whether that's maintaining current weight or losing some if needed. Together, they act as a protective shield against many of the adverse consequences of menopause, while at the same time laying the foundation for lifelong strength, energy, and disease prevention.

While the primary focus of this book is nutrition, it would be a disservice not to include exercise. Nutrition and exercise are a one-two punch, and if you want the best chances of securing a knockout, that's a winning combination. Exercise is critical when it comes to transitioning through menopause. Not only can exercise help alleviate some of your symptoms, it can help increase your energy and positively impact your body's internal chemistries, thus having a tremendous impact on your overall health. I'm not suggesting that you need to exercise for hours a day and live in a gym, rather I'm suggesting that the work you do by eating smarter will be enhanced when you exercise smarter and consistently.

An essential part of your workout plan needs to be resistance training (free weights, machines, resistance bands) that leads to building more muscle. Cardio is still important and should be done, but muscle building is critical during menopause. A tremendous amount of research has consistently shown that overall health can be improved when you increase or preserve your muscle mass and improve your muscle-to-fat ratio. After the age of thirty, women begin to lose between 3 percent and 8 percent of their muscle mass each decade, and this loss accelerates dramatically during and after menopause. This phenomenon of muscle loss (which also occurs with men as they age) is known as sarcopenia and leads to decreased physical strength, compromised mobility, poor balance, and a slower metabolism. Estrogen helps preserve muscle mass by influencing how amino acids (the small building blocks of proteins, which are the building blocks of muscle) are used in the body. As estrogen declines, resistance training becomes one of the most effective ways to counteract its loss. By lifting weights, using resistance bands, working out with machines, or performing bodyweight exercises, women stimulate muscle protein synthesis, which helps preserve and rebuild lean tissue.

In addition to helping maintain strength and physical independence, muscle also plays a crucial role in metabolic health. Muscle is metabolically active tissue, meaning it burns calories even at rest. The more muscle a woman has, the higher her resting metabolic rate (RMR), which determines how many calories she burns throughout the day. This becomes critically important during menopause, because a sluggish metabolism—partly driven by hormonal shifts and muscle loss—makes it easier to gain weight even when eating the same types and quantities of food that didn't previously cause weight gain. By actively building and maintaining muscle, women can counteract this metabolic slowdown and improve their body's ability to burn fat.

Resistance training is also one of the most effective lifestyle interventions for protecting bone health. Estrogen plays a pivotal role in maintaining bone density, and its decline during and after menopause puts women at heightened risk for osteoporosis and fractures. Strength training, particularly weight-bearing movements like squats, deadlifts, and lunges, sends signals to the bones to strengthen and rebuild themselves. Over time, this process improves bone mineral density, reduces the risk of fractures, and helps maintain good posture and spinal health, all things that are especially important as women age.

Another powerful benefit of building muscle is its ability to improve insulin sensitivity. As estrogen levels fall, many women become more insulin resistant, which means the important functions that insulin serves become diminished, and this can lead to higher blood sugar levels and increased risk of type 2 diabetes. The body always needs the right amount of insulin at the right time to be able to control the levels of sugar in the blood. Muscle helps regulate blood glucose by drawing sugar from the bloodstream and then using it as fuel. This improved metabolic function means better blood sugar regulation, less inflammation, and improved cardiovascular health.

It's also important to note that regular resistance training positively influences mental and emotional well-being. Exercise releases natural feel-good chemicals like endorphins, reduces cortisol, and improves levels of brain-derived neurotrophic factor (BDNF), which supports cognition and memory—two areas that can be affected during menopause. Endorphins serve a variety of functions, including alleviating pain, lowering stress, enhancing your sense of well-being, and improving mood. They are created and released by the brain when you do activities that are pleasurable, like exercising, creating art, getting a massage, or watching a TV show that you enjoy. Cortisol is called the stress hormone, because it's released in response to various stressors (running late for work, getting into a car accident, someone attempting to hit you) that you might encounter. While some cortisol is necessary during stressful times, too much of this hormone over a prolonged period of time can be counterproductive and cause symptoms such as weight gain (especially around the face and abdomen), thinning skin, fatigue, elevated blood pressure, and mental health challenges such as increased irritability and anxiety and difficulty concentrating. Exercise can alleviate and potentially prevent some of these symptoms by lowering cortisol levels.

Weight loss—especially fat loss—is the other big reason why building muscle becomes even more critical as we age. As estrogen declines, many women begin to experience a redistribution of fat, particularly around the midsection. This visceral fat, which accumulates around internal organs, is more than just a potential aesthetic concern—it is metabolically harmful. Visceral fat is linked to chronic inflammation and significantly raises the risk of cardiovascular disease, type 2 diabetes, insulin resistance, and certain cancers such as breast and endometrial cancer. For women who are overweight, losing even a modest amount of weight, such as 5–10 percent of total body weight, can lead to dramatic improvements in health markers like blood pressure, cholesterol, fasting blood glucose, and inflammation levels.

Maintaining and/or achieving a healthy weight during menopause is also critical for lowering systemic inflammation. Fat tissue isn't just passive storage, rather it's biologically active and secretes pro-inflammatory cytokines. These compounds can worsen joint pain and fatigue and even exacerbate autoimmune conditions. When women lose weight—especially by reducing fat stores—they lower these inflammatory signals, which can lead to improved energy, reduced joint pain, and a decrease in brain fog.

Fat loss also plays a significant role in balancing hormones. Fat cells produce estrone, a weaker form of estrogen that can interfere with the body's hormonal signaling. During menopause, excess fat can further disrupt the balance between estrogen, progesterone, and insulin, worsening symptoms like hot flashes, night sweats, mood swings, and fatigue. By reducing excess fat, women create a more stable internal environment that supports better hormone regulation and fewer symptoms.

In addition to the internal benefits, weight loss significantly improves physical function. Carrying extra weight creates a burden on the joints, particularly the knees and hips, which increases the risk of osteoarthritis and limits mobility. Every extra ten pounds of body weight above a healthy weight (BMI has traditionally been the guide for determining healthy weight; however, that measurement has come under scrutiny recently, so check with your healthcare provider) can put an additional thirty to sixty pounds of pressure on the joints during activity. By reducing weight, women reduce this mechanical stress, which not only relieves pain but also enables them to be more active and engaged in daily life.

Beyond the physical, both muscle building and fat loss have enormous psychological payoffs. As women see their strength increase and their bodies change, confidence in their bodies and their mental well-being soar.[24] They experience better sleep, enhanced libido, sharper mental focus, and more emotional resilience. These changes contribute to a greater sense of control and empowerment during a life stage that can often feel uncertain or overwhelming.

Importantly, muscle building and weight loss must be pursued together. Focusing solely on weight loss without preserving or increasing muscle mass can result in a slower metabolism and higher likelihood of regaining the weight. Likewise, building muscle without managing body composition may not reduce the health risks associated with excess fat. Together, these two goals form a synergistic strategy—building muscle preserves metabolism and function, while weight loss improves hormone balance and reduces disease risk. The result is a stronger, leaner, more vibrant body that is equipped to not only handle menopause, but thrive well into the decades beyond it.

DON'T WASTE TIME IN THE GYM

Many people have good intentions when they enter a gym or begin an exercise program. However, a lack of understanding of what exercises to do or how to do them means they are not getting the most out of their workouts and are not making the most of their time. Gym management and workout efficiency are important and should be stressed. Busy people don't have time to waste doing unnecessary workouts that deliver little bang for the buck. There's no reason why exercise can't be fun, but it should also be productive.

One of the best ways to be efficient with your workouts is to have a plan. You should know what you are going to do and why you are doing it before you begin each exercise session. Goals are also important, and not just general goals, but specific goals. "I want to build more muscle" is very different than "I want to build more muscle strength in my arms, shoulders, and legs." Having direction gives your workouts purpose and practicality and prevents you from working out aimlessly with few results to show for all of your hard work.

We all have different goals for different reasons, but at the top of the list should be muscle growth and retention and preserving joint health. According to celebrated national trainer Joey Thurman, author of *The Minimum Method*, "Different areas of the body such as the glutes and hips should come into focus as women age. These areas are crucial for posture, pelvic control, and joint health—and tend to weaken with age."

A good trainer, even if you engage one for just a short period of time, can make a huge difference. They can help you develop a plan, teach you which exercises are best for you, and show you proper lifting form and techniques that will keep you safe and help you get the most out of your workouts. Not everyone has the budget for a trainer, of course, so don't be discouraged in the least if you're in a similar financial position. There are thousands of great instructional videos online that can help you better understand what you need to do and how to do it. Take advantage of free online resources from credible sources and start building a plan that addresses the specific goals that you have established. You can also use the following blueprint I have created as a starting point.

THE PLAN

The exercise plan in this chapter is meant to be a foundation upon which you can design and build a workout strategy that best suits your needs and goals. It's virtually impossible to create a single plan that will work for everyone, so I have structured this one in a way that provides a solid platform upon which to build a customized routine that works for you.

This four-week program can be repeated and built on with each iteration. Following the detailed program are lists of exercises that can be done for each of the major muscle groups. There is also a list of cardiovascular exercise options that you can do with and without machines. You can choose the exercises you want from the list or from outside the list and substitute them into the plan for similar exercises so that it's customized for you. There is total flexibility to make it easier for you. What is not flexible is that you must do something and you must do it consistently. Even if you can't do the full 40 minutes, do 15 or 20 minutes. You can also break the session into two sessions—one in the morning and the other in the afternoon or at night. However you decide to do it is fine, as long as you put in the work, because it's the consistency and the challenge you put your body under that are going to deliver results!

Most days have a corresponding QR code that can be used to watch a video demonstration of the exercises. There are also videos for some of the alternate exercises listed at the end of this chapter. As with any exercise program, always consult a healthcare professional and fitness trainer to make sure it's safe for you to follow and that you are doing the exercises correctly. When reading the exercise instructions, note that the first number in the exercise is the amount of sets you are supposed to do and the second number is the number of repetitions in each set. For example, 3 x 12 means 3 sets of 12 repetitions. In weeks 2 through 4, the number of repetitions are just suggestions. Do as many reps as you can, until you can't complete a rep using good form.

High-intensity interval training (HIIT) is a specific workout method that alternates between short bursts of intense activity and brief periods of rest or low-intensity movement, for example, 30 seconds of fast-paced exercise (like sprinting or jumping jacks) followed by 30–60 seconds of rest or gentle movement, then repeat the cycle. It is an extremely popular and effective exercise strategy, and I've included it in the exercise plan.

HIIT is a particularly beneficial exercise approach because it delivers maximum results in minimal time. It boosts heart rate, increases calorie burn, and improves both cardiovascular fitness and metabolic health—even after the workout ends (a phenomenon known as the "afterburn effect"). For women in menopause, HIIT can be especially beneficial for:

- Burning visceral fat.
- Improving insulin sensitivity.
- Enhancing cardiovascular endurance.
- Boosting mood and energy.

Since most HIIT workouts take just 20 to 30 minutes, they are a time-efficient way to improve health, lose weight, and build lean muscle without long hours in the gym.

Tips for HIIT success in menopause:

- Keep intervals short and intense (20–40 seconds of work, 40–60 seconds of rest).
- Aim for six to ten total cycles, depending on fitness level.
- Take 5–10 minutes to warm up before and cool down after each session.
- Include at least one to two HIIT sessions per week to boost cardiovascular health, insulin sensitivity, and fat loss.

WEEK 1 (3 DAYS)

Day 1: Full-Body Strength (Upper + Lower)

Goblet Squats: 3 sets x 12 reps
Dumbbell Chest Presses: 3 x 10
Bent-Over Rows: 3 x 12
Standing Core Twists: 3 x 15

Day 3: Cardio (Steady State)

Brisk walking, elliptical, or cycling: 30–40 minutes at a moderate pace

Day 5: Lower-Body Strength (Glutes + Hamstrings)

Glute Bridges: 3 x 15
Dumbbell Deadlifts: 3 x 10
Standing Calf Raises: 3 x 20
Side Lunges: 3 x 10/leg

WEEK 2 (4 DAYS)

Day 1: Upper-Body Strength (Back + Biceps)

Dumbbell Rows: 3 x 12
Bicep Curls: 3 x 10
Lat Pulldowns or Band Pulls: 3 x 12
Seated Russian Twists: 3 x 20

Day 3: Cardio (HIIT)

5 rounds: 40 seconds work / 20 seconds rest (choose to jog, jump rope, or bike sprint)

Day 4: Lower-Body Strength (Quads + Glutes)

Step-Ups: 3 x 10/leg
Dumbbell Squats: 3 x 12
Wall Sits: 3 x 30 seconds

Day 6: Core + Mobility

Planks: 3 x 30 seconds
Bird Dogs: 3 x 15/side
Dynamic Stretching/Yoga: 15–20 minutes

WEEK 3 (5 DAYS)

Day 1: Upper-Body Strength (Chest + Triceps)

Push-Ups (wall/floor): 3 x 10
Tricep Dips: 3 x 12
Chest Flys: 3 x 12

Day 2: Cardio (Steady State)

Outdoor walking or stationary cycling at a steady pace: 40 minutes

Day 3: Lower-Body Strength (Glutes + Core)

Hip Thrusts: 3 x 12
Leg Raises: 3 x 15
Side Planks: 2 x 30 seconds/side

Day 5: Cardio (HIIT)

6 rounds: 30 seconds work / 30 seconds rest (choose sprints, stairs, or fast walking—treadmill optional; or bike)

Day 6: Full-Body Recovery Flow

Foam Rolling + Yoga Sequence: 30 minutes

WEEK 4 (5 DAYS)

Day 1: Lower-Body Strength (Quads + Glutes)

Goblet Squats: 3 x 12
Walking Lunges: 3 x 10/leg
Glute Kickbacks (bands or machine): 3 x 15/leg
Standing Calf Raises: 3 x 20

Day 2: Cardio (Steady State)

Brisk walking, incline treadmill, or swimming laps at a steady pace: 35–40 minutes

Day 3: Upper-Body Strength (Shoulders + Back)

Dumbbell Shoulder Presses: 3 x 10
Upright Rows: 3 x 12
Reverse Flys: 3 x 15
Renegade Rows (light weight): 3 x 8/side

Day 5: Cardio (HIIT)

For all HIIT workouts with multiple exercises: One option is to do the specified number of rounds of one exercise (here, five), followed by that number of rounds of the second exercise, followed by the same number of rounds of the third exercise. The other option is to do the exercises sequentially per round. You would do the first exercise for 30 seconds, then rest for 30 seconds, followed by the second exercise for 30 seconds, then rest for 30 seconds, followed by the third exercise for 30 seconds. That would complete round one. You would rest for a full minute, then repeat the same sequence for round two. Keep going until you complete the specified number of rounds.

5 rounds: 30 seconds work / 30 seconds rest

- High Knees
- Jump Squats or Step Jacks
- Mountain Climbers

Rest 1 minute between rounds.

Day 6: Core + Recovery Stretch

Plank Holds: 3 x 30 seconds
Leg Lowers: 3 x 15
Supine Twist + Cobra Stretch + Forward Fold: 3 rounds of deep breathing

ADDITIONAL EXERCISES

The list of exercises that follow are here for you to use at your discretion; they can be substituted into the suggested four-week exercise plan anytime you want. They provide you with lots of options so you can vary your workout and choose exercises that best fit your abilities and goals, customizing your plan to best fit your needs.

CARDIOVASCULAR AND BODYWEIGHT EXERCISES

HIIT Exercises with Machines

1. **Treadmill Sprints or Incline Walks**
   Sprint or walk fast for 30 seconds, then rest for 30–60 seconds.
2. **Elliptical Surges**
   Push hard for 40 seconds at high resistance, then recover for 20 seconds.
3. **Rowing Machine Intervals**
   Row as fast as possible for 20–30 seconds, then recover at a slower pace for 60 seconds.
4. **Stationary Bike Sprints**
   Cycle hard for 30 seconds, then switch to easy pedaling for 60 seconds.
5. **Stair Climber Intervals**
   Climb quickly for 45 seconds, then slow down for 45 seconds.
6. **Battle Ropes**
   Slam or wave ropes intensely for 20 seconds, then rest for 40 seconds.
7. **SkiErg Machine Sprints**
   Pull powerfully for 30 seconds, then slow down or rest for 60 seconds.

HIIT Exercises Without Machines (Bodyweight or Light Equipment)

1. **Jump Squats**
   Do explosively for 20 seconds, then rest for 40 seconds. (Modify with bodyweight squats for joint sensitivity.)
2. **Mountain Climbers**
   Do at a brisk pace for 30 seconds, then rest for 30 seconds.
3. **High Knees**
   Run in place, driving knees high, for 20 seconds, then rest for 30–60 seconds.
4. **Jumping Jacks or Step Jacks**
   Do 30 seconds of jumping jacks or step jacks, then rest for 30 seconds. (Step jacks are a low-impact version of jumping jacks where you step out instead of jumping.)
5. **Lateral Skaters**
   Do side-to-side lunges with a hop for 30 seconds, then rest for 30 seconds.
6. **Punch-Outs with Light Dumbbells**
   Jab fast in front of you while holding light weights for 20–30 seconds, then rest for 30 seconds.
7. **Plank Jacks**
   From a plank position, jump feet out and in for 20–30 seconds, then rest for 30 seconds.
8. **Ice Skaters**
   Mimic the side-to-side motion of speed skating for 30 seconds, then rest for 30 seconds.

RESISTANCE (STRENGTH) TRAINING

Chest Exercises (Pectorals)

1. **Push-Ups** (wall, incline, or floor)
2. **Chest Presses** (dumbbells or machine)
3. **Chest Flys** (dumbbells or cable)
4. **Incline Chest Presses** (dumbbells)
5. **Incline Chest Flys**
6. **Resistance Band Chest Presses**
7. **Cable Crossovers** (upper-chest focus)
8. **Stability Ball Dumbbell Presses**
9. **Single-Arm Dumbbell Chest Presses**
10. **Isometric Wall Chest Presses** (press palms against a wall in front of the chest for 20–30 seconds)

Biceps Exercises

1. **Bicep Curls** (dumbbells)
2. **Hammer Curls** (neutral grip to hit forearms, too)
3. **Resistance Band Curls**
4. **Concentration Curls**
5. **Cable Bicep Curls**
6. **EZ Bar Curls**
7. **Incline Dumbbell Curls**
8. **21s Bicep Curls**
9. **Zottman Curls**
10. **Isometric Curl Holds** (hold at 90 degrees for 30 seconds)

Triceps Exercises

1. **Tricep Dips** (chair or bench)
2. **Overhead Tricep Extensions** (dumbbell or band)
3. **Tricep Kickbacks** (dumbbells)
4. **Close-Grip Push-Ups**
5. **Skull Crushers** (lying tricep extensions)
6. **Tricep Pushdowns** (cable or band)
7. **Single-Arm Overhead Extensions**
8. **Reverse Grip Tricep Pushdowns**
9. **Resistance Band Tricep Presses**
10. **Isometric Wall Pushes with Bent Elbows**

Shoulder Exercises (Deltoids)

1. **Shoulder Presses** (dumbbells or bands)
2. **Lateral Raises** (to the side)
3. **Front Raises** (straight in front)
4. **Arnold Presses** (rotational press)
5. **Rear Delt Flys** (reverse flys)
6. **Upright Rows** (dumbbells or band)
7. **Overhead Band Pull-Aparts**
8. **Face Pulls** (cable or band)
9. **Single-Arm Overhead Presses**
10. **Plank to Down Dog Shoulder Activation**

Core Exercises (Abs, Obliques, Lower Back)

1. **Planks** (forearm or high)
2. **Bird Dogs**
3. **Dead Bugs**
4. **Russian Twists** (bodyweight or light weight)
5. **Leg Raises** (lying on back)
6. **Bicycle Crunches**
7. **Side Planks** (with knee down or straight legs)
8. **Seated Knee Tucks** (on chair or floor)
9. **Flutter Kicks**
10. **Standing Oblique Crunches**

Glute Exercises (Gluteus Maximus, Medius, Minimus)

1. **Glute Bridges**
2. **Hip Thrusts** (on bench or floor)
3. **Donkey Kicks**
4. **Fire Hydrants**
5. **Step-Ups**
6. **Bulgarian Split Squats** (rear foot elevated)
7. **Resistance Band Lateral Walks**
8. **Single-Leg Glute Bridges**
9. **Glute Kickbacks** (with or without cable/band)
10. **Frog Pumps**

Quadriceps Exercises

1. **Squats** (bodyweight or dumbbell)
2. **Walking Lunges**
3. **Wall Sits**
4. **Step-Ups** (quad-dominant)
5. **Leg Extensions** (machine)
6. **Split Squats** (stationary)
7. **Front Foot Elevated Lunges**
8. **Sissy Squats** (supported if needed)
9. **Seated Knee Extension Isometric Holds**
10. **Chair Squats**

4-Week Menopause Exercise Plan

Week	Day	Workout Type	Exercises
1	1	Full-Body Strength (Upper + Lower)	• Goblet Squats: 3x12 • Dumbbell Chest Presses: 3x10 • Bent-Over Rows: 3x12 • Standing Core Twists: 3x15
1	3	Cardio (Steady State)	• Brisk walking, elliptical, or cycling: 30–40 mins at moderate pace
1	5	Lower-Body Strength (Glutes + Hamstrings)	• Glute Bridges: 3x15 • Dumbbell Deadlifts: 3x10 • Standing Calf Raises: 3x20 • Side Lunges: 3x10/leg
2	1	Upper-Body Strength (Back + Biceps)	• Dumbbell Rows: 3x12 • Bicep Curls: 3x10 • Lat Pulldowns or Band Pulls: 3x12 • Seated Russian Twists: 3x20
2	3	Cardio (HIIT)	• 5 rounds: 40 secs work / 20 secs rest (jog, jump rope, or bike sprint)

Week	Day	Workout Type	Exercises
2	4	Lower-Body Strength (Quads + Glutes)	• Step-Ups: 3x10/leg • Dumbbell Squats: 3x12 • Wall Sits: 3x30 secs
2	6	Core + Mobility	• Planks: 3x30 secs • Bird Dogs: 3x15/side • Dynamic Stretching/Yoga: 15–20 mins
3	1	Upper-Body Strength (Chest + Triceps)	• Push-Ups (wall/floor): 3x10 • Tricep Dips: 3x12 • Chest Flys: 3x12
3	2	Cardio (Steady State)	• Outdoor walking or stationary cycling: 40 mins at steady pace
3	3	Lower-Body Strength (Glutes + Core)	• Hip Thrusts: 3x12 • Leg Raises: 3x15 • Side Planks: 2x30 secs/side

Week	Day	Workout Type	Exercises
3	5	Cardio (HIIT)	• 6 rounds: 30 secs work / 30 secs rest (sprints, stairs, fast walking, or bike)
3	6	Full-Body Recovery Flow	• Foam Rolling + Yoga Sequence: 30 mins
4	1	Lower-Body Strength (Quads + Glutes)	• Goblet Squats: 3x12 • Walking Lunges: 3x10/leg • Glute Kickbacks: 3x15/leg • Standing Calf Raises: 3x20
4	2	Cardio (Steady State)	• Brisk walking, incline treadmill, or swimming laps: 35–40 mins at steady pace
4	3	Upper-Body Strength (Shoulders + Back)	• Dumbbell Shoulder Presses: 3x10 • Upright Rows: 3x12 • Reverse Flys: 3x15 • Renegade Rows: 3x8/side

Week	Day	Workout Type	Exercises
4	5	Cardio (HIIT)	• 5 rounds: 30 secs work / 30 secs rest • High Knees • Jump Squats or Step Jacks • Mountain Climbers • Rest 1 min between rounds
4	6	Core + Recovery Stretch	• Plank Holds: 3x30 secs • Leg Lowers: 3x15 • Supine Twist + Cobra Stretch + Forward Fold: 3 rounds

6

REAL WOMEN, REAL RESULTS

There comes a moment in every woman's journey—sometimes quiet, sometimes overwhelming—when she realizes that her body no longer responds the way it used to. The same meals now lead to weight gain. The energy she once counted on to get through her day has vanished. And no matter how many products, diets, or routines she tries, nothing seems to work quite like it used to.

This chapter is about that moment, and what happens when women choose to rise above it. For many women, menopause can feel like a slow unraveling of their identity. The weight gain is frustrating, yes, but the deeper impact is often invisible—the unpredictable moods, the sleepless nights, the shame that builds when your body feels unfamiliar. Too often, women are told to just "deal with it." It's normal. It's just age. It's inevitable. The truth, however, is that while menopause is natural, suffering through it isn't. There are real tools, rooted in science, that can help you feel strong, clearheaded, and grounded in your body again. And the proof of that doesn't come from perfect influencers or unrealistic before-and-after photos you might see on social media. It comes from real women who are dealing with real-life challenges, just like you.

In the following pages, you'll meet six women who once stood in the same place you and millions of other women are—overwhelmed, frustrated, and on the verge of giving up. They had tried countless diets. They battled many of the common symptoms like hot flashes, mood swings, bloating, brain fog, and joint pain. They felt lost in a maze of conflicting advice. But when they began to work *with* their bodies and not *against* them, everything changed.

These women didn't follow fad diets or go to trendy extremes. Instead, they embraced a new approach—a menopause-smart lifestyle that prioritized anti-inflammatory foods, balanced their blood sugar, optimized hormonal support, and focused on consistent movement and exercise. More importantly, they committed to *progress, not perfection*. They found sustainable habits that respected their time, budget, and emotional bandwidth.

The results were AMAZING:

- 15 to 25 pounds lost.
- Blood pressure and cholesterol lowered.
- Joint pain and night sweats eased.
- Energy, mood, and sleep restored.
- A new sense of empowerment gained and self-trust reclaimed.

Perhaps most beautiful of all, these women reconnected with themselves. They began to enjoy cooking again. They moved their bodies in joyful, pain-free ways. They found confidence not because they became someone new, but because they remembered who they'd always been.

This chapter isn't just about celebrating transformation; it's about showing you what's possible when you're given a plan that finally works *with* your hormones in this unique stage of life. If you've ever wondered if you're just "too far gone," felt invisible or alone in your menopause journey, or wished for proof that it really *can* get better, then these stories are for you. Let these women show you that change is not only possible, but absolutely within your reach. Their journeys might just help rewrite your own.

LINDA—THE CORPORATE EXEC WHO FOUND HER ENERGY AGAIN

Age: 52
Location: Dallas, Texas
Starting Weight: 186 lbs
10-Week Weight Loss: 18 lbs

Linda, a high-powered HR executive, was always in control until menopause hit. Hot flashes during boardroom meetings left her embarrassed, and brain fog made her second-guess her instincts. "I felt like I was melting down at my desk," she said.

Linda had long prided herself on her ability to multitask and make quick decisions to lead teams. But menopause blindsided her. The very skills she had honed over decades of leadership seemed to suddenly unravel overnight. Frustrated by sudden mood swings and a sense of disconnection from her body, she knew something had to change. Her typical morning started with coffee and takeout—habits that had once sustained her fast-paced lifestyle but were now contributing to inflammation, energy crashes, and disrupted sleep.

After consulting with her doctor, Linda committed to a structured anti-inflammatory menopause plan focused on lean proteins, healthy fats, leafy greens, and phytoestrogens like flaxseed and soy. She reduced sugar, limited caffeine, and increased hydration. She also began daily walks to clear her mind and establish a rhythm for her day. The first thing she noticed was that within a few weeks, the fog began to lift. She then noticed her energy returning, her sleep improving, and even her skin regaining some of its glow.

What began as a desperate attempt to regain control evolved into a complete transformation. Today, Linda not only manages her symptoms, but leads her company's new wellness initiative, helping other women find their own path through menopause. Her story is proof that menopause doesn't have to derail your life—instead, it can redirect you toward a stronger, wiser, and more vibrant version of yourself.

What Worked

Linda thrived with structure. The plan's detailed daily breakdown of meals and snacks appealed to her Type A personality and busy calendar, because it allowed her to create an effective meal prep system. By planning and cooking on Sundays, she removed the mental load of making decisions during her hectic workdays. The new diet helped reduce cortisol spikes, which are linked to increased belly fat during menopause.

She made sure her diet was rich in omega-3 fatty acids (from foods like salmon, walnuts, and chia seeds), which help modulate inflammation and reduce the severity of hot flashes. She also included phytoestrogens (like in flaxseeds, soy, and chickpeas), which bind to estrogen receptors in the body and help mimic the effects of declining estrogen, improving thermoregulation and mood.

One of her most challenging tasks was reducing refined sugars and caffeine, which can trigger hot flashes and amplify anxiety. She swapped in green tea and herbal infusions that gave her the antioxidants she needed without overstimulating her system. Linda's body responded quickly to the consistency, and her focus sharpened within weeks.

Exercise Approach

Linda's schedule has been hectic for years; however, she was determined to make room for exercise, because she knew how important it was in helping her alleviate symptoms and gain better control of her health. She started with twenty-minute power walks during lunch and added two brief evening resistance band workouts per week. "I kept it simple with just a mat, my bands, and some music. It fit right into my routine without stressing me."

By week four, her mental clarity returned, and the frequency of her hot flashes dropped from multiple daily episodes to just once or twice per week. By week ten, she'd lost eighteen pounds, rediscovered her energy, and regained her professional confidence. "I'm not fighting my body anymore. I'm finally supporting it."

Habit Transformation

Habit #1: Skipping Meals → Structured, Nourishing Meals

Before: Linda's schedule was so packed that she often skipped breakfast and lunch, only to overeat late at night when she got home. This pattern created unstable blood sugar levels and increased her cortisol—a double whammy during menopause, when hormonal regulation is already compromised.

After: Using *The New Menopause Kitchen*'s meal plan, Linda began eating something for breakfast even if it was light, batch cooking on Sundays, and portioning out protein-rich salads, soups, and stir-fries she could easily grab throughout the week. Eating a protein- and fiber-rich lunch by 1 PM daily helped stabilize her insulin, which reduced cravings and reduced her tendency to overeat in the evenings. She also reported fewer energy dips throughout the day and felt more mentally alert in meetings.

Habit #2: Overreliance on Caffeine → Strategic Hydration with Green Tea and Water

Before: Like many people, Linda drank coffee not necessarily because she enjoyed the taste of it, but rather what it did for her. Her daily four to five cups would help her power through exhaustion, especially after nights of poor sleep. While caffeine can boost your energy in the short term, in high doses it can worsen anxiety, sleep disturbances, and hot flashes during menopause.

After: Linda knew this was going to be a habit that would take time to change. She made a plan to gradually taper her consumption and finally got down to one morning cup of coffee and replaced her afternoon doses with decaffeinated iced green tea, which contains L-theanine—a calming compound that improves focus without increasing cortisol. She also committed to drinking half her body weight in ounces of water per day, often infused with lemon, cucumber, or mint. This helped her stay hydrated, reduced hot flashes, and improved skin tone and digestion.

Reflection Prompts: From Burnout to Balance

Linda's story is a powerful reminder that even the most capable, accomplished women can feel unsteady when menopause hits. Her identity as a leader, decision-maker, and problem-solver didn't disappear—it simply needed new support. By giving her body structure, nourishment, and space to breathe, she didn't just survive menopause—she used it as a launching pad for personal and professional renewal. Take a few minutes to check in with yourself.

If you paused right now and asked your body what it needs, what would it say? Examples: rest, hydration, movement, real food, quiet, forgiveness.

What does "structure" look like for you? What kind of routine could help reduce stress and decision fatigue? Examples: meal prepping, scheduled breaks, daily movement, a planned evening wind-down.

What old habits have been hard to let go of even though they may no longer serve you? Examples: skipping meals, relying on caffeine to get through the day, working through lunch, fast-food dinners, late-night screen time.

In what ways has menopause (or perimenopause) disrupted your daily rhythms or performance? Examples: brain fog in meetings, irritability with coworkers or family, low energy during the day, lack of motivation to work out.

Linda learned to lead herself before leading others again. What would it mean for you to support your body instead of fighting it? What's one step you could take this week to shift from burnout to balance?

MELISSA—THE EMPTY NESTER WHO DITCHED BLOATING AND BAGGAGE

Age: 55
Location: Los Angeles, California
Starting Weight: 172 lbs
10-Week Weight Loss: 16 lbs

When Melissa sent her youngest child off to college, she imagined a new chapter as an empty nester filled with freedom and rediscovery. The idea of having the house to herself, time to travel, and no more late-night school projects felt like a long-awaited reward. But once the quiet settled in, something unexpected happened—she felt lost and without purpose.

Rather than basking in her newfound independence, Melissa felt physically uncomfortable and emotionally unmoored. Her body, once predictable, now seemed foreign to her. She started experiencing problems with her digestion, feeling bloated after meals with frequent gas and unpredictable bowel movements. Foods she once tolerated now left her feeling heavy and inflamed. Her waistline noticeably expanded, and no matter how much she cut back on portions, the scale wouldn't budge. "It felt like my body had completely changed overnight," she recalled.

Emotionally, she was on a roller coaster. Some days she felt numb and unmotivated; others, she snapped at her partner for no obvious reason. The sudden waves of sadness, irritability, and restlessness left her questioning whether she was truly entering a new chapter or simply falling apart. She felt like she had become a different person. "I thought once the kids were gone, I'd finally feel free. But instead, I felt like I was disappearing into someone I didn't recognize."

Though she had always tried to maintain a positive body image when things weren't always looking or feeling the way she wanted, nothing in her previous experience had prepared her for this version of herself. She now found herself in midlife, menopausal, and unbalanced in body and mind. She started searching for answers, desperate to regain control not just of her weight, but of her sense of self. She was given early access to *The New Menopause Kitchen*, and that's when she came across the concept of gut-centered healing during menopause—an approach that connected the dots between hormonal shifts, inflammation, digestion, and mood. It resonated with her immediately. "No one had ever told me that my gut and hormones were talking to each other," she said. "But it made so much sense. I realized I had to stop punishing my body and start helping it heal."

What Worked

Melissa's primary struggles—bloating, digestive discomfort, and mood swings—were addressed by a diet rich in prebiotics, probiotics, and anti-inflammatory spices. Fermented foods like kefir, sauerkraut, and miso introduced beneficial bacteria to her gut that improved her microbiome diversity and reduced systemic inflammation.

She made good use of prebiotic fiber, especially from some of her favorite foods—asparagus, oats, and bananas. They helped feed those healthy gut microbes, which improved her digestion and serotonin production, both key for mood regulation. Foods like turmeric and ginger helped soothe her gut lining and reduce post-meal discomfort.

Melissa paid close attention to the section of the plan that addressed the benefits of removing inflammatory triggers like refined wheat, excess dairy, and alcohol. This significantly reduced intestinal irritation and allowed her body to absorb nutrients more effectively. Increased hydration helped improve her digestion and reduced water retention. These simplified but highly strategic changes brought about a rapid turnaround in her overall digestive health and led to more emotional stability and less physical discomfort.

Exercise Approach

With her newfound time, Melissa joined a neighborhood walking group three times a week. "The community made it easy to stick with it." Even though the plan called for scheduled rest days, she decided to do something on those days, too—beginner Pilates she learned on YouTube. She was engaging in something called "active recovery," low-intensity exercise that helps the body recover from previous high-intensity exertion. She said, "I liked the Pilates, because it was gentle and made my body feel supported."

Her bloating disappeared by week five, and by week ten, she'd lost sixteen pounds, her digestion was smoother, and she felt emotionally lighter. "This was about more than food. It was about finally letting go of what wasn't serving me."

Habit Transformation

Habit #1: Evening Wine and Cheese → Gut-Friendly Alternatives

Before: After dinner, Melissa often unwound with wine and cheese, which became her emotional outlet as she adjusted to an empty home. However, both alcohol and dairy can increase inflammation, disrupt digestion, and worsen mood swings in menopausal women.

After: Melissa swapped wine for sparkling water with a splash of tart cherry juice or kombucha—both of which support digestion and have antioxidant benefits. She also substituted probiotic-rich hummus, kimchi, or kefir yogurt for cheese. This shift drastically reduced her bloating and helped improve her gut-brain connection, boosting serotonin production and regulating her mood.

Habit #2: All-Day Grazing → Three Mindful Meals + Occasional Snacks

Before: With less structure in her day, Melissa found herself grazing constantly—nuts here, crackers there. She was eating when she wasn't even hungry, just because the food was there or she was looking for something to do. This led to sluggish digestion and overeating.

After: She adopted a pattern of three balanced meals, each with a focus on lean protein, fiber, and healthy fats, plus one intentional snack if needed. This stabilized her blood sugar, enhanced her feeling of fullness, and gave her digestion time to rest between meals. She also began eating more slowly and without watching TV or looking at her phone, and this helped her become more mindful and enjoy meals with less stress.

Reflection Prompts: Reclaiming Your Midlife Balance

Melissa's story is a powerful reminder that menopause isn't just about physical changes—it's also about redefining your relationship with yourself. As her gut healed, her energy returned and her mood stabilized, with her confidence quietly reawakened. Take a few minutes to reflect on your own experience.

What physical changes have you noticed in your body over the last six to twelve months? Examples: bloating, weight gain, fatigue, food sensitivities, joint pain.

If you could feel *just one* positive shift in your body over the next ten weeks, what would it be? Examples: more energy, better digestion, looser clothes, steadier moods.

What habits—nutritional or emotional—do you sense are no longer serving you well? Examples: late-night snacking on sweets, turning to food when stressed, excessive worry about things not in your control.

How have changes you've made affected your mood, confidence, or daily life? Examples: less irritability, more confidence, increased motivation, greater desire to socialize.

What is one small, realistic step you can take this week to begin healing from the inside out—just like Melissa did? Examples: try one gut-friendly meal, swap a snack, add a probiotic food, take a ten-minute post-meal walk.

LORETTA—THE ENTREPRENEUR WHO GOT HER GLOW BACK

Age: 46
Location: Atlanta, Georgia
Starting Weight: 213 lbs
10-Week Weight Loss: 25 lbs

Loretta had always been a powerhouse and fearless. She built her clothing boutique from the ground up—juggling payroll, managing a team of young stylists, and overseeing inventory—all while raising teenage twins and maintaining a fierce sense of style and independence. Her friends called her "the woman who never stops moving." She seemed to have boundless energy and could stretch a twenty-four-hour day into twenty-five.

All of this seemed to change in her mid-forties. Without warning, she quickly began gaining weight. First it was five pounds, then ten, and then twenty, all concentrated around her waist and hips. Her once thick, shiny hair began to thin along her temples. She noticed a drop in energy and found herself unable to get through her workday without feeling extremely tired. She even fell asleep a few times in the middle of the day. The way she treated her kids changed, too. She snapped at them over things that never used to faze her. Worst of all, the spark she had always carried—the spark that lit up her store and her home—felt like it was fading.

"I didn't recognize myself anymore," Loretta said. "I wasn't just tired. I was disconnected from my body, my joy, even my creativity."

She tried to "push through" like she always had in the past. She cut calories, did YouTube workout challenges at 5 AM, skipped meals, and drank more coffee to give herself a boost. However, regardless of what she did, her body refused to budge. "The things that used to work just didn't anymore," she said. "It was like my body had changed the lock, and I didn't have the new key."

At first, she thought maybe she was just burned out, but when the hot flashes started—suddenly, violently, right in the middle of helping a customer zip up a dress—she realized it was more than that. Her mood swings became more intense, and her sleep—when she could sleep at all—was broken and shallow. "One day I looked in the mirror and thought, *My God, this isn't just stress. This is menopause.*"

Determined to regain control, Loretta began researching approaches to support her body through this hormonal transition. She jumped at the chance to try the *New Menopause Kitchen* program, excited to hear that it was possible to alleviate some of her symptoms not through medications, but through a hormone-smart eating plan designed specifically for midlife women. It emphasized foods that nourished her hormones and reduced inflammation, all without requiring her to count calories or deprive herself.

What Worked

The plan's emphasis on hormone-friendly nutrition to combat early menopause symptoms like weight gain, fatigue, and thinning hair registered with her. She incorporated zinc- and iron-rich plant proteins (like lentils, quinoa, pumpkin seeds, and black beans), which supported thyroid function and energy production—both crucial during hormonal shifts.

She started drinking daily smoothies that included flaxseeds and cruciferous vegetables (spinach, kale, broccoli), which can provide plant-based phytoestrogens. These ingredients help balance estrogen metabolism and improve skin health. The convenience and portability of this new smoothie ritual and its clear effects on her mood, energy, and skin made it easy for her to stay consistent, even during long workdays.

As suggested by the plan, Loretta also avoided added sugars and soda to lower her inflammation and improve her insulin sensitivity—a major factor in weight loss during menopause. Her hydration-focused routine, including herbal teas and lemon water, helped flush toxins and improve skin clarity.

By week five, her skin brightened and mood improved. By week ten, she was down twenty-five pounds and saw hair regrowth around her hairline. "I couldn't believe how much better I felt, and I got my glow back."

Exercise Approach

With a packed schedule, Loretta committed to "ten-minute minimums." She did short HIIT workouts or dance breaks in her office. "Sometimes I'd put on music and dance with my employees between customers—it counted!" On weekends, she walked or biked with her kids. She got her ten minutes in six days a week and varied her activity to keep it interesting.

Habit Transformation

Habit #1: Skipping Breakfast → Energizing Morning Smoothie Ritual

Before: Loretta often skipped breakfast due to her busy mornings, leading to fatigue and intense sugar cravings by mid-afternoon. Skipping meals during menopause can disrupt blood sugar and cortisol rhythms, contributing to irritability, fatigue, and weight gain.

After: She began each day with a hormone-balancing smoothie made with flaxseed, kale, almond milk, berries, vegan protein powder, and avocado. This gave her sustained energy, stabilized her appetite, and gave her skin a noticeable glow. Even when she had only five minutes in the morning, the ease and portability made her smoothie ritual sustainable.

Habit #2: Snacking Mindlessly at Work → Movement Breaks as Mood Boosters

Before: Loretta often grazed between client appointments, grabbing chips, chocolate, or pastries to deal with boredom or stress. Whatever was within reach, she grabbed it. She nibbled almost constantly throughout her workday.

After: She set hourly timers for five-minute movement breaks, when she would walk around the store, do light stretching, or turn on a favorite playlist and dance with her staff. These "micro workouts" helped regulate her blood sugar, reduce cravings, and elevate her mood. She also began packing portion-controlled snacks like a healthy, low-sugar trail mix, fruit, and protein bars to eat mindfully.

Reflection Prompts: Rediscovering Your Spark

Loretta's story is a reminder that menopause isn't the end of vitality, rather it's an invitation to reconnect with your power, nourish your body with intention, and redefine what strength and beauty look like in this season of life. Her journey started not with restriction, but with *respect*—for her hormones, her energy, and her evolving needs. Take a few minutes to reflect on your own experience.

In what ways do you feel like you've "lost your spark" lately—physically, emotionally, or creatively? Be honest and gentle. This is a space for noticing, not judging.

What would it feel like to let go of the pressure to be perfect and instead focus on *progress and consistency*?

What does "getting your glow back" mean to you personally? Examples: feeling lighter in your body, feeling confident in your clothes, having energy to enjoy your day.

What are you doing in your daily routine that *may* be dimming your glow? Examples: skipping meals, over-caffeinating, not moving, eating in a rush.

What's one small way you can start nourishing yourself again—like Loretta did with her morning smoothie ritual? Examples: prepping a veggie-packed lunch, walking ten minutes after dinner, drinking herbal tea instead of soda.

EMILY—THE TEACHER WHO RECLAIMED HER SLEEP AND SANITY

Age: 48
Location: Detroit, Michigan
Starting Weight: 205 lbs
10-Week Weight Loss: 22 lbs

Emily had always been the kind of teacher who lit up a room. With over two decades in the classroom, she was known for her patience, creativity, and ability to reach even the most challenging students. Her days were spent organizing lesson plans, guiding curious minds, and managing the beautiful chaos that comes with teaching middle schoolers. But in the year leading up to her forty-ninth birthday, everything began to change—and not in ways she had expected.

First came the insomnia. Nights once filled with deep, restorative sleep turned into restless tossing and turning, followed by unexplained 3 AM wakeups with racing thoughts. Then came the night sweats. She would soak through her pajamas and sheets, forcing her to change clothes in the dark before dragging herself through the rest of the night. The exhaustion piled up, and with it came irritability and a rising sense of anxiety that began to seep into her workday.

"I was angry, exhausted, and felt like my body hated me," Emily shared. "I'd always been the steady one, the calm one, and now I was snapping at students, forgetting where I put my attendance sheets, and crying for no good reason in the staff bathroom during lunch."

Emily began skipping workouts and grabbing fast food more often—not out of laziness, but purely for survival. "I had no energy to cook, let alone think about what I was eating. I just wanted to get through the day." As her weight began creeping up, her self-esteem went sliding down. The mental fog, bloating, and unpredictable emotions all felt like an ambush.

Yet every time she tried to seek help, she was met with vague reassurances and told that this was just part of getting older.

Something inside her—perhaps the same quiet strength that made her such a resilient educator—refused to accept that this was just her "new normal." One afternoon, while researching menopause symptoms between classes, Emily stumbled across an article that linked sleep disruption, frequent urination and fatigue (due to blood sugar instability), and muscle spasms and cramps (due to magnesium deficiency) to perimenopause. It was the first time she saw her symptoms explained in a way that made sense and, more importantly, gave her hope.

She saw a social media post looking for volunteers to try a new plan focused on helping menopausal women by restoring balance through food and not restriction. She signed up and received an early draft of *The New Menopause Kitchen*, which emphasized magnesium-rich foods to calm the nervous system, complex carbs to regulate cortisol, and plant-based proteins to support hormone metabolism. Miracles weren't promised, but the plan offered something better: a gentle, sustainable way forward.

"I wasn't looking for perfection," Emily said. "I just wanted to feel like myself again."

What Worked

Emily decided to prioritize magnesium-rich foods to help calm her nervous system and improve her sleep quality. Magnesium plays a critical role in GABA production (a neurotransmitter that promotes relaxation) and supports the body's stress response—especially important for women facing perimenopausal anxiety and insomnia.

She also reduced her consumption of refined sugars and focused on eating complex carbohydrates like quinoa, oats, and sweet potatoes to stabilize her blood sugar and prevent nighttime glucose crashes that can trigger cortisol spikes and night sweats.

One of her favorite rituals—a nightly tea routine—acted as both a physical and psychological wind-down cue, and became her sanctuary. "Drinking my chamomile and magnesium tea before bed felt nurturing," she said. This consistent behavior helped regulate her circadian rhythm. "It helped me finally sleep."

Emily also cut back on processed snacks in favor of nutrient-dense options like hummus, seed crackers, and sliced cucumbers, which kept her satisfied without the roller coaster of energy dips. By improving her nutrition and creating calming rituals, Emily significantly reduced sleep disruption and emotional irritability within just a few weeks.

Exercise Approach

Emily began reintroducing exercise to her day with restorative yoga in the evenings. "Just fifteen minutes helped me release tension." As her energy returned, Emily added morning walks before school twice a week. "I needed something quiet and grounding."

By week four, her night sweats had nearly disappeared. By week ten, she'd lost twenty-two pounds, was sleeping well, and felt emotionally balanced for the first time in years. "Menopause doesn't have to mean misery. You just have to give your body the right tools."

Habit Transformation

Habit #1: Nighttime Snacking → Soothing Evening Wind-Down Ritual

Before: Exhausted after a full day of teaching, Emily frequently reached for chips, cookies, or sweet cereal before bed. These foods spiked her blood sugar, leading to disrupted sleep, night sweats, and increased belly fat.

After: She replaced nighttime snacks with a wind-down routine that included herbal tea (chamomile or magnesium-based), light stretching, and screen-free time. This helped lower her cortisol and prepare her nervous system for rest. By sticking to a consistent 9:30 PM sleep ritual, her night sweats drastically decreased, and within four weeks she was sleeping through the night again.

Habit #2: Emotional Eating at Work → Prepared Anti-Inflammatory Snacks

Before: Midday stress at school led Emily to raid the break room for sugary or processed snacks, which made her feel even more fatigued and irritable once her sugar high crashed.

After: She began packing anti-inflammatory snacks such as almond butter packets, roasted chickpeas, sliced cucumbers, seed crackers, and small portions of 70 percent dark chocolate to eat instead. These options provided steady energy without spiking her blood sugar, and gave her the sense of control she needed during overwhelming moments. She kept them in her desk drawer along with herbal stress drops and a water bottle to reinforce hydration.

Reflection Prompts: Restoring Rest and Reclaiming Calm

Emily's story is one many women can relate to. When her sleep fell apart, so did her energy, her mood, and her sense of self. But through small, steady changes—adding calming foods and routines, and deciding to prioritize her well-being—she reclaimed her rest, her patience, and her power. Take a moment to reflect on your own relationship with rest, recovery, and nourishment.

How would you describe your sleep over the past few months? Examples: broken, light, delayed, nonexistent. Do you wake up tired even after a full night?

What habits or routines might be contributing to your current sleep challenges? Examples: late-night screens, sugar or caffeine too late in the day, eating too close to bedtime.

What are three words that describe how you *feel* during the day as a result of your sleep? Examples: edgy, foggy, flat, wired, overwhelmed, anxious, resigned.

If you could do one thing tonight to support deeper, restorative sleep, what would it be? Examples: warm herbal tea before bed, lights off by 10 PM, no phone in bed, reading instead of scrolling, deep breathing, a magnesium-rich snack like almonds or pumpkin seeds.

ASHLEY—THE NURSE WHO BALANCED HER HORMONES AND HER LIFE

Age: 50
Location: Charlotte, North Carolina
Starting Weight: 194 lbs
10-Week Weight Loss: 20 lbs

Ashley was no stranger to long hours, stress, or the unpredictable demands of caring for others. As a veteran night-shift nurse in a busy trauma unit, she had learned how to thrive in chaos. She could stay calm during emergencies, think fast on her feet, and comfort families in crisis—all while running on very little sleep and a strong cup of coffee. But when she turned fifty, something changed. And for the first time in her career, it wasn't a shift she could manage or a symptom she could diagnose away.

It started subtly—aching joints that lingered longer, knees that creaked after a twelve-hour shift, weight gain that came out of nowhere despite no change in her diet. Her period, once regular and predictable, became erratic and intense. She'd go months without one, only to be hit with what felt like a flood while on the job, leaving her exhausted and anxious. Her moods fluctuated without warning, and she found herself waking up drenched in sweat after barely two hours of broken sleep.

"I was used to being tired," she said. "But this wasn't tired. This was being totally drained. This was foreign to me. I felt like I was aging in fast-forward and couldn't hit pause."

Ashley had always prided herself on being strong and composed, but now even the smallest things overwhelmed her. She snapped at coworkers, forgot simple details, and began dreading her shifts. "I was taking care of everyone else's emergencies, but no one was taking care of mine—including me."

She tried going back to the gym but found it too exhausting. She cut calories but saw no change. The health advice she knew so well no longer seemed to apply to the woman in the mirror. "I kept wondering how I could know so much about health and still feel so out of control in my own body."

Then, during a late shift, she read a medical journal article on the impact of night shifts on hormonal balance in menopausal women, and something clicked. For the first time, her symptoms weren't just random; they were connected. Her disrupted circadian rhythm, poor sleep hygiene, and erratic eating patterns were throwing her hormones even further off track. That insight became her turning point.

Ashley began researching menopause-specific strategies and discovered information that suggested it was possible to support hormone balance through nutrition, especially for women who work irregular hours. She learned how certain foods—particularly those rich in magnesium, calcium, vitamin D, and omega-3s—could help restore hormonal harmony. She also adopted intermittent fasting, adjusting her meals to align better with her sleep-wake cycle instead of eating heavy meals during her overnight shifts.

"It was the first time I felt like I had a strategy," she said. "I wasn't fighting my body anymore. Instead, I was supporting it."

What Worked

Ashley's plan was built around bone-supportive, anti-inflammatory nutrition to address her joint pain and hormone fluctuation. She prioritized calcium- and magnesium-rich vegetables like kale, bok choy, and broccoli, along with vitamin D from mushrooms, egg yolks, and fortified almond milk. These nutrients are critical to preserving bone density and supporting neuromuscular function during menopause. Ashley regularly drank collagen-rich bone broth, which supports joint health and reduces inflammation in connective tissues. She also included anti-inflammatory fats like avocado, walnuts, and fatty fish to help ease her joint pain.

By using intermittent fasting and avoiding late-night meals during shifts, Ashley supported her digestive rhythm and allowed her insulin levels to stabilize, something that's critical for fat metabolism and hormonal balance. "When I stopped eating late, my digestion calmed down." The timed eating window was surprisingly effective. "It gave me boundaries." The flexibility of the *New Menopause Kitchen* plan, which allowed her to eat nutrient-dense foods during her "feeding window," was key to making the plan sustainable with her unpredictable schedule.

After just seven weeks, Ashley was excited to report that her hormonal symptoms, weight, and energy levels all improved after adopting nutritional strategies that targeted both her lifestyle and her metabolic needs.

Exercise Approach

Ashley used a flexible "movement menu." On workdays, she stretched after shifts. On her days off, she went for nature walks or did yoga. "If I had ten minutes, I moved. If I had thirty, I danced or did weights. No guilt."

By week six, her joints ached less. By week ten, she was twenty pounds lighter and was able to return to activities she loved without any pain. "This diet wasn't a restriction. It was a rescue plan."

Habit Transformation

Habit #1: Eating During Night Shifts → Time-Restricted Feeding Aligned with Her Circadian Rhythm

Before: Ashley had spent years eating her "dinner" at 2 AM in the hospital break room, usually something quick and heavy like pasta, a sandwich, or fast food picked up from the drive-through on her way in. She often followed that with heavy snacking to stay awake. This pattern disrupted her blood sugar, spiked cortisol, and interfered with melatonin production, making it harder for her to sleep after her shift.

After: Ashley transitioned to a time-restricted feeding window that better matched her body's natural rhythm. She ate her main meals during the daytime—starting with a balanced breakfast before going to sleep once she got home, followed by lunch when she woke up and a lighter early dinner before heading to work. During her overnight shifts, she sipped on herbal tea and occasionally had a small, digestive-friendly snack like cucumber slices with hummus or a boiled egg—nothing too heavy. This reduced the burden on her digestive system, improved her sleep quality, and helped regulate insulin and cortisol levels. She also noticed fewer cravings and more energy during her shift now that she was off the blood sugar roller coaster.

Habit #2: Overexertion and Inconsistent Workouts → Short, Restorative Movement She Could Handle Consistently

Before: In the past, Ashley believed a workout had to be intense and sweaty to count. She tried pushing herself to do HIIT workouts and spin classes after her shifts, but they just left her depleted and sore. As her joint pain increased, she gave up entirely, feeling defeated. "I thought if I couldn't do a *real workout*, it wasn't worth doing," she said.

After: Ashley replaced that all-or-nothing mindset with a gentler, more consistent movement plan. She began doing short mobility routines and yoga flows on her off days, focusing on joint support, circulation, and flexibility. During her shifts, she built in intentional walking breaks (even just ten minutes between rounds) and added resistance band strength training twice a week at home. These low-impact exercises helped reduce inflammation, strengthen her muscles, and relieve the stiffness that had once kept her off her feet. More importantly, the realistic schedule made it sustainable. "Movement became medicine, not punishment," she said. "And that's what made it stick."

Reflection Prompts: Finding Balance in a Demanding Life

Ashley's story shows that even when life is nonstop—when you're caring for others, working long hours, and barely getting any rest—*you can still reclaim balance.* Her transformation wasn't about working harder. It was about working *with* her body instead of against it.

Now it's your turn to reflect on how your current habits are supporting—or straining—your hormones.

What part of Ashley's journey resonates most with you? Is it letting go of perfection? Eating with intention? Shifting from burnout to balance?

How do you currently move your body throughout the week? Is your movement all or nothing? Too intense? Nonexistent due to time or fatigue?

What is one form of gentle movement you could add that feels restorative instead of exhausting? Examples: walking outside for fifteen minutes, stretching your arms and legs then walking in place for five minutes, single-leg alternating balance exercises.

Do your meals match your natural energy patterns? Are you eating heavy meals at night? Skipping breakfast? Snacking through the evening?

What's one change you could make to better align your eating with your body's rhythm? Examples: eating more protein on days you do strength training, eating a lighter dinner when you are forced to eat late, cutting your calories by 10 percent for every ten pounds of weight you lose.

BECKY—THE SKEPTIC WHO FINALLY FOUND WHAT WORKED

Age: 57
Location: Kansas City, Missouri
Starting Weight: 198 lbs
10-Week Weight Loss: 15 lbs

Becky had always considered herself someone who followed the rules, and she applied that in all aspects of her life, including when it came to eating. She read food labels, watched her portions, and made an effort to stay informed about nutrition trends. Over the years, she had rotated through nearly every diet she could find—low-carb, keto, Mediterranean, intermittent fasting, even a cabbage soup cleanse she saw on TikTok that promised it would "reset everything." But despite all the effort, all the tracking, and all the restraint, her weight wouldn't budge.

"I felt like I was being punished for trying," she said. "I'd lose two pounds one week and gain back three the next. No matter what I did, it never stuck. I started to think my metabolism was just broken."

Each year, her cholesterol levels were also creeping higher. When her doctor raised the red flag during her annual checkup, gently mentioning the word "statins," it hit Becky harder than she expected. "I remember sitting in the parking lot afterward thinking, *Is this it? Is this just what happens now? Is there nothing I can do?*"

But weight and labs weren't her only struggles. Becky had been quietly dealing with persistent joint stiffness, especially in the morning. Her energy was flat, and she often needed a nap just to get through the afternoon. What bothered her most was the underlying sense that she was slipping further and further away from the woman she used to be—sharp, vibrant, and in control of her body.

"I'd look in the mirror and think, *I still feel young in my head*. But my body was telling a different story. I wasn't ready to give up, but I didn't know what else to try."

What finally changed the game was a conversation with a friend from her book club who had recently gone through a menopause-specific nutrition program. The friend looked vibrant—lighter not just in body but in spirit. Becky was skeptical at first, assuming it was just another restrictive diet in disguise. But her friend insisted: "This isn't about cutting more. It's about giving your body what it's been missing."

Intrigued and out of options, Becky decided to give it one last try. She wanted a plan that didn't demonize food or demand perfection, rather one that focused on nourishing her hormones, reducing chronic inflammation, and stabilizing blood sugar—all with everyday ingredients she could find at her local grocery store. She looked at the structure and meal plan of *The New Menopause Kitchen* and thought it would be a good fit.

After completing the ten weeks, Becky said, "It seemed completely different from everything else I'd tried. I wasn't starving. I wasn't obsessing. I was feeding myself in a way that made me feel steady both physically and emotionally."

What Worked

What shocked Becky wasn't only how effective the plan was, but how simple and affordable it was. "I didn't have to buy fancy powders or overpriced supplements," she said. "Just real food I could get at my grocery store."

She learned how to cook easy, five-ingredient meals like turmeric-spiced lentils, roasted chickpeas with sweet potatoes, and one-pan salmon with broccoli. The anti-inflammatory meal options made grocery shopping a breeze—mostly fresh produce, frozen veggies, affordable whole grains like brown rice and oats, and plant-based proteins.

She began enjoying cooking again—something she hadn't done since her kids moved out. "I put on music and made it fun," she said. "And I couldn't believe how much better I felt just eating real, colorful food." For Becky, the simplicity of the recipes was one of the plan's biggest gifts. She didn't have to count macros or track calories.

Exercise Approach

A lifelong "non-exerciser," Becky started walking twenty minutes a day, mostly in the evenings after dinner. "That was all I could commit to at first. But the more energy I had, the more I wanted to move." By week six, she was doing light yoga and short strength circuits at home with resistance bands she had purchased many years ago but had never used.

Habit Transformation

Habit #1: Ordering Takeout Most Nights → Cooking Simple, Affordable Meals at Home

Before: Becky had fallen into the habit of ordering takeout or picking up premade meals most nights. "It felt easier after a long day," she admitted. But this convenience came at a cost. Most of the meals she ordered were high in saturated fat, sodium, and refined carbohydrates, which contributed to her elevated cholesterol and stubborn weight. Even salads came drenched in sugary dressings or with fried toppings. The habit also had become expensive and left her feeling guilty.

After: Becky reframed cooking as self-care and not another source of stress. She began with no-fuss, thirty-minute recipes that required minimal ingredients. She even customized the plan by creating a simple formula for her meal planning that she followed not all the time, but often:

- 1 lean protein (beans, eggs, tofu, or fish)
- 1 healthy fat (avocado, olive oil, or nuts)

- 1 complex carb (brown rice, lentils, or sweet potato)
- Unlimited non-starchy veggies (spinach, cauliflower, or Brussels sprouts)

Batch cooking on Sundays became a ritual, and she used leftovers creatively throughout the week. By prepping staples ahead of time (like roasted vegetables, hard-boiled eggs, and cooked grains), she could throw together meals in under ten minutes.

Habit #2: Being Sedentary All Day → Adding Daily Low-Impact Movement

Before: Becky's days were mostly sedentary. She worked from home and didn't prioritize physical activity. After dinner, she'd often go straight to the couch to unwind, sometimes watching TV until late at night, before finally sliding into bed and falling asleep next to her husband. This lack of movement contributed to joint stiffness, weight gain, and a general sense of heaviness and fatigue.

After: Becky started small by committing to post-dinner walks around her neighborhood. "It helped with digestion and gave me time to clear my mind," she said. She eventually added short yoga sessions she found on YouTube, which helped ease the chronic tension in her hips and back, and a gentle strength circuit. She was surprised at how much she enjoyed working out, and discovered the exercises improved her circulation, muscle tone, and joint mobility.

Reflection Prompts: From Frustration to Freedom

Becky's story is one many women know all too well—trying everything and getting nowhere. So much about weight maintenance in a changing body can be overwhelming, whether it's the exhaustion of chasing results, the heartbreak of feeling like your body is failing you, or the fear that maybe nothing will ever work. But Becky's breakthrough came when she stopped punishing her body and started nourishing it instead. Now it's your turn to reflect.

How might your body be trying to communicate with you right now? What are your symptoms (for example, fatigue, bloating, pain, mood swings, cravings) trying to tell you?

What diets or food rules have you tried in the past that left you feeling frustrated or restricted? Did they work temporarily? Did they help or harm your relationship with food or your body?

What messages have you internalized over the years about weight gain, menopause, or your worth? Examples: "I have no discipline," "This is just aging," "I'm broken," "I'll never lose weight again."

What would "steady and sustainable" look like for you in this season of life? Think beyond the scale. Examples: better blood lab results, fewer symptoms, more energy, increased confidence, emotional calm.

What's one change you could make in how you eat or care for yourself to help you shift, like Becky did, from restriction to nourishment? Examples: eat three real meals a day, add greens to your plate, cook more at home, hydrate more often.

Moving Forward: Nourishment, Strength, and the New You

Menopause is not a period of decline, rather it's a biological turning point that's an invitation to rewrite the narrative of what health and vitality look like in midlife and beyond. The drivers of this narrative are strategic nutrition and targeted exercise.

What you put on your plate becomes a daily act of empowerment. Anti-inflammatory, whole-food-based eating isn't just about symptom management—it's about building your resilience. A diet rich in leafy greens, omega-3 fatty acids, plant-based phytoestrogens, lean proteins, and high-fiber foods can help stabilize hormones, reduce chronic inflammation, improve gut health, and protect against postmenopausal risks like cardiovascular disease, osteoporosis, and metabolic slowdown. Each meal is an opportunity to nourish your changing body with intention.

Equally transformative is movement. Whether it's a brisk walk, strength training, swimming, or yoga, physical activity strengthens bones, enhances mood, improves metabolic health, and preserves cognitive function. Resistance training, in particular, is one of the most effective ways to combat age-related muscle loss and bone density decline—two of the most pressing health risks for postmenopausal women. The benefits of exercise go beyond the physical. Consistent and determined exercise is proven to reduce stress, improve sleep quality, and elevate confidence.

Together, food and movement are not to be viewed as restrictive mandates, but rather as regenerative medicine. They support you in not just "getting through" menopause, but in thriving during it. Keep reminding yourself that you are not losing your power—you are reclaiming it. Every step you take and every nourishing bite you eat send a message to your body: You are still vital. You are still strong. You are still evolving.

Most importantly, even during the most difficult times, don't forget that this journey is yours. There is no one-size-fits-all formula for menopause, so dedicate your energy to making informed, intentional choices that honor your unique needs, values, and goals. Whether you're just entering perimenopause or are navigating life after menopause, it's never too late to reset your habits and reclaim your health. You deserve to feel vibrant, strong, and whole. With knowledge, support, and consistency, the path ahead is not only manageable—it can be enjoyable, renewing, and deeply empowering.

Appendix I: Life-Changing Recipes

The following recipes created by my good friend Rachael Ray have been designed specifically for you. They are simple, delicious, fortifying, and full of powerful nutrients. While they can be incorporated into the ten-week meal plan, as shown in chapter four, they are also designed as stand-alone meals to help you better customize your menopause-friendly diet.

Be adventurous and try as many of them as you can. If you need to substitute some of the ingredients, by all means feel free to do so. Rachael is the first one to say that the kitchen is like a laboratory, where you should feel free to experiment and explore and make the recipes and ingredients your own. It's ideal to use fresh and unprocessed ingredients; however, just do the best you can within your budget, your physical capabilities, and whatever you have available.

Most importantly, have fun with these recipes. Use them to build new recipes. And share them with family members or friends; these delicious recipes are suitable for everyone. Good food is here for us to savor, share, and enjoy. Happy eating!

BREAKFAST

Almond Butter and Banana Smoothie

Servings: 1

1 medium banana
2 tablespoons almond butter
1 cup unsweetened almond milk
1 tablespoon chia seeds
1 teaspoon honey (optional)

Combine all the ingredients in a blender and blend until smooth.

Nutritional Information (per serving): *Calories: 320; Protein: 9g; Carbohydrates: 36g; Fat: 18g; Fiber: 6g*

Apple Cinnamon Oatmeal

Servings: 2

1 cup rolled oats
2 cups water or milk
1 medium apple, cored and diced
1 teaspoon ground cinnamon
1 tablespoon honey or maple syrup (optional)

1. In a small saucepan, combine the oats, water, apple, and cinnamon. Bring to a boil, then reduce the heat and simmer for 5 to 7 minutes, until the oats are cooked.
2. Stir in the honey or maple syrup, if desired.

Nutritional Information (per serving): *Calories: 230; Protein: 6g; Carbohydrates: 42g; Fat: 4g; Fiber: 6g*

Avocado Toast with Tomato and Egg

Servings: 1

½ medium avocado, peeled, pitted, and mashed
1 slice whole-grain bread, toasted
1 tomato, sliced
1 large egg, hard-boiled, peeled, and sliced
1 teaspoon extra-virgin olive oil (optional)
Salt and pepper to taste

Spread the mashed avocado on the toast. Layer with the tomato and hard-boiled egg slices. Drizzle with olive oil (if using) and season with salt and pepper.

Nutritional Information (per serving): *Calories: 300; Protein: 11g; Carbohydrates: 26g; Fat: 18g; Fiber: 8g*

Berry Oatmeal Bake

Servings: 4

2 cups rolled oats
2 cups unsweetened almond milk
½ cup fresh blueberries
½ cup fresh raspberries
¼ cup maple syrup
1 teaspoon vanilla extract
1 teaspoon ground cinnamon
½ teaspoon baking powder

1. Preheat the oven to 350°F (175°C). Lightly grease a small baking dish.
2. In a medium bowl, mix all the ingredients until well combined.
3. Pour into the prepared baking dish and bake for 25 to 30 minutes, until set.

Nutritional Information (per serving): *Calories: 220; Protein: 6g; Carbohydrates: 39g; Fat: 5g; Fiber: 6g*

Chia Seed Pudding with Berries

Servings: 2

¼ cup chia seeds
1 cup unsweetened almond milk
1 tablespoon maple syrup (optional)
1 cup mixed fresh berries (such as strawberries, blueberries, raspberries)

1. In a bowl, whisk together the chia seeds, almond milk, and maple syrup (if using). Let sit in the fridge for at least 4 hours or overnight.
2. Serve topped with the mixed berries.

Nutritional Information (per serving): *Calories: 230; Protein: 6g; Carbohydrates: 32g; Fat: 10g; Fiber: 14g*

Greek Yogurt Parfait

Servings: 2

1 cup nonfat or low-fat Greek yogurt
½ cup granola
1 cup mixed fresh berries (such as strawberries, blueberries, raspberries)
1 tablespoon honey (optional)

In two glasses or small bowls, layer half of the yogurt, granola, and berries. Drizzle each serving with half of the honey, if desired.

Nutritional Information (per serving): *Calories: 300; Protein: 20g; Carbohydrates: 45g; Fat: 6g; Fiber: 5g*

Overnight Oats with Almonds and Apples

Servings: 1

½ cup rolled oats
1 cup unsweetened almond milk
½ medium apple, cored and diced
2 tablespoons raw almonds, chopped
1 teaspoon ground cinnamon
1 tablespoon maple syrup (optional)

In a jar or bowl, combine all the ingredients and mix well. Cover and refrigerate overnight. Enjoy cold in the morning.

Nutritional Information (per serving): *Calories: 290; Protein: 8g; Carbohydrates: 40g; Fat: 12g; Fiber: 6g*

Savory Oatmeal with Spinach and Eggs

Servings: 2

2 cups vegetable broth
1 cup rolled oats
1 cup chopped fresh spinach
2 large eggs
1 tablespoon nutritional yeast (optional)
Salt and pepper to taste

1. In a small saucepan, bring the vegetable broth to a boil. Add the oats and cook according to the package instructions. Stir in the spinach until wilted.
2. In a separate pan, poach or fry the eggs.
3. Serve the oatmeal topped with the eggs, and sprinkle with the nutritional yeast (if using), salt, and pepper.

Nutritional Information (per serving): *Calories: 320; Protein: 16g; Carbohydrates: 40g; Fat: 10g; Fiber: 6g*

Sweet Potato and Kale Frittata

Servings: 6

2 tablespoons extra-virgin olive oil
2 medium sweet potatoes, peeled and diced
2 cups chopped kale
6 large eggs
Salt and pepper to taste
¼ cup crumbled feta cheese

1. Preheat the oven to 375°F (190°C).
2. In an oven-safe skillet, heat the olive oil over medium heat. Add the sweet potatoes and cook, stirring often, until tender, 20 to 30 minutes. Add the kale and cook, stirring, just until wilted.
3. In a bowl, whisk together the eggs, salt, and pepper. Pour over the sweet potatoes and kale. Top with the feta.
4. Cook, stirring often, until the eggs are mostly set, 2 to 3 minutes. Transfer the skillet to the oven and bake for 15 to 20 minutes, until fully set.

Nutritional Information (per serving): *Calories: 200; Protein: 12g; Carbohydrates: 18g; Fat: 10g; Fiber: 3g*

Tristé's Bone Density Smoothie

Servings: 1

¾ cup plain full-fat kefir or Greek yogurt
5 prunes (or 4 medium plums), pitted
½ cup fresh or frozen blueberries
½ small banana (optional; for sweetness and potassium)
1 ½ tablespoons ground flaxseed
1 tablespoon hemp seeds
Pinch of cinnamon
¼ cup of water or unsweetened almond milk

1. Add the kefir or yogurt to a blender, followed by the prunes, blueberries, banana (if using), ground flaxseed, and hemp seeds. Then add the cinnamon and liquid.
2. Blend for 30–45 seconds or until smooth.
3. Drink immediately, as flaxseeds oxidize over time.

Nutritional Information (per serving): *Calories: 371; Protein: 25g; Carbohydrates: 64g; Fat: 13g; Fiber: 10g*

LUNCH AND DINNER

Aglio e Olio

Servings: 6

½ cup extra-virgin olive oil
10 anchovy fillets, drained
8 garlic cloves, minced
1 tablespoon Calabrian chili paste
½ cup dry vermouth
1 pound dried spaghetti
1 cup chopped fresh flat-leaf parsley
Juice of 1 small lemon
Pinch of salt for water boiling

1. Bring a large pot of salted water to a boil for the pasta.
2. Meanwhile, heat the olive oil in a large, deep skillet with a lid over medium heat. Add the anchovies and gently mash them into the oil with a wooden spoon or flat wooden paddle. (The anchovies will melt into the oil and no longer taste fishy; they will taste more like salted nuts!) Add the garlic, chili paste, and vermouth and stir to combine. Reduce the heat to low and cover the pan.
3. Add the spaghetti to the boiling water and cook a minute shy of the package instructions (to allow for carry-over cooking). Transfer 1 cup of the pasta cooking water to the sauce in the skillet, then drain the pasta and add it to the sauce, along with the parsley and lemon juice.

Nutritional Information (per serving): *Calories: 510; Protein: 13g; Carbohydrates: 50g; Fat: 27g; Fiber: 2g*

Baked Chicken with Vegetables

Servings: 4

2 cups chopped mixed vegetables (such as carrots, zucchini, bell peppers)
2 tablespoons extra-virgin olive oil, divided
1 tablespoon dried Italian seasoning
Salt and pepper to taste
4 (6-ounce) boneless, skinless chicken thighs
Juice of 1 lemon

1. Preheat the oven to 400°F (200°C).
2. In a large bowl, toss the mixed vegetables with 1 tablespoon of the olive oil, the Italian seasoning, salt, and pepper.
3. Place the chicken thighs in a small baking dish and drizzle with the lemon juice and remaining 1 tablespoon olive oil. Season with salt and pepper. Add the vegetables around the chicken in the baking dish.
4. Bake for 25 to 30 minutes, until the chicken is cooked through and the vegetables are tender.

Nutritional Information (per serving): *Calories: 280; Protein: 25g; Carbohydrates: 10g; Fat: 15g; Fiber: 3g*

Baked Salmon with Asparagus

Servings: 4

4 (4-ounce) salmon fillets
1 bunch asparagus, woody ends snapped off
2 tablespoons extra-virgin olive oil
Salt and pepper to taste
1 lemon, sliced

1. Preheat the oven to 400°F (200°C). Line a rimmed baking sheet with parchment paper.
2. Arrange the salmon and asparagus on the prepared baking sheet. Drizzle with the olive oil and season with salt and pepper. Top with the lemon slices.
3. Bake for 15 to 20 minutes, until the salmon is cooked through.

Nutritional Information (per serving): *Calories: 280; Protein: 28g; Carbohydrates: 6g; Fat: 16g; Fiber: 2g*

Beet and Quinoa Salad

Servings: 2

1 cup cooked quinoa
1 cup diced roasted beets
¼ cup crumbled feta cheese
¼ cup walnuts, chopped
2 tablespoons extra-virgin olive oil
1 tablespoon apple cider vinegar
Salt and pepper to taste

1. In a large bowl, combine the quinoa, beets, feta, and walnuts.
2. In a small bowl, whisk together the olive oil, vinegar, salt, and pepper.
3. Drizzle the dressing over the salad and toss gently.

Nutritional Information (per serving): *Calories: 380; Protein: 9g; Carbohydrates: 32g; Fat: 26g; Fiber: 7g*

Caprese Salad with Avocado

Serves: 4

2 large tomatoes, sliced
1 medium avocado, peeled, pitted, and sliced
1 cup sliced fresh mozzarella
¼ cup fresh basil leaves
2 tablespoons balsamic glaze
1 tablespoon extra-virgin olive oil
Salt and pepper to taste

Arrange the tomato, avocado, and mozzarella slices on a plate, alternating them. Sprinkle with the basil leaves, drizzle with the balsamic glaze and olive oil, and season with salt and pepper.

Nutritional Information (per serving): *Calories: 250; Protein: 10g; Carbohydrates: 12g; Fat: 20g; Fiber: 4g*

Cauliflower Rice Stir-Fry

Servings: 4

2 tablespoons toasted sesame oil
2 garlic cloves, minced
1 head cauliflower, riced, or 4 cups refrigerated or frozen cauliflower rice
1 cup chopped mixed vegetables (such as carrots, peas, bell peppers)
2 tablespoons soy sauce or tamari
Sliced scallions, for garnish

In a large skillet, heat the sesame oil over medium heat. Add the garlic and stir-fry for 30 seconds. Add the cauliflower rice and mixed vegetables and stir-fry for 5 to 7 minutes, until tender. Stir in the soy sauce and cook for 1 minute. Garnish with scallions.

Nutritional Information (per serving): *Calories: 150; Protein: 5g; Carbohydrates: 12g; Fat: 10g; Fiber: 4g*

Chicken and Quinoa Bowl

Servings: 4

2 tablespoons extra-virgin olive oil, divided
2 (6-ounce) boneless, skinless chicken breasts, cut into bite-size pieces
Salt and pepper to taste
2 cups cooked quinoa
1 cup cherry tomatoes, halved
1 cucumber, diced
½ cup crumbled feta cheese
1 tablespoon balsamic vinegar
Chopped fresh flat-leaf parsley, for garnish

1. In a large skillet, heat 1 tablespoon of the olive oil over medium heat. Add the chicken, season with salt and pepper, and cook, stirring occasionally, until browned and cooked through, 7 to 10 minutes.
2. Transfer the chicken to a large bowl and add the quinoa, cherry tomatoes, cucumber, and feta. Drizzle with the remaining 1 tablespoon olive oil and the balsamic vinegar. Toss gently to combine and garnish with parsley.

Nutritional Information (per serving): *Calories: 350; Protein: 30g; Carbohydrates: 30g; Fat: 14g; Fiber: 3g*

Chicken in Salsa Verde

Servings: 4

Sauce

½ (28-ounce) can poblano peppers, stemmed, seeded, and drained
½ (28-ounce) can crushed tomatillos
4 garlic cloves, crushed
1 small onion, chopped
½ cup fresh cilantro
Juice of 2 limes
1 tablespoon ground cumin
1 teaspoon dried oregano
Salt and pepper to taste

Chicken

4 (6-ounce) chicken cutlets
Salt and pepper to taste
3 tablespoons extra-virgin olive oil
1 (28-ounce) can black beans, rinsed, drained, and warmed
2 cups cooked brown rice

1. Combine all the sauce ingredients in a blender and puree; set aside.
2. Season the chicken liberally on both sides with salt and pepper. Heat the olive oil in a large nonstick skillet over medium heat. Add the chicken and brown the first side for a few minutes, then turn and lightly brown the other side for another few minutes.

3. Add the sauce to the skillet, turn the heat down to medium-low, and simmer for about 15 minutes to thicken a bit.
4. Serve the chicken and sauce with the black beans and brown rice.

Nutritional Information (per serving): *Calories: 430; Protein: 31g; Carbohydrates: 45g; Fat: 16g; Fiber: 8g*

Coconut Curry Chicken

Servings: 4

2 tablespoons extra-virgin olive oil
1 pound boneless, skinless chicken thighs, cut into bite-size pieces
1 tablespoon grated fresh ginger
2 garlic cloves, minced
1 tablespoon curry powder
1 (14-ounce) can coconut milk
1 cup sliced bell peppers (any color)
1 cup chopped fresh spinach
Salt and pepper to taste

1. In a large skillet, heat the olive oil over medium heat. Add the chicken and cook, stirring often, until browned, 5 to 7 minutes. Stir in the ginger, garlic, and curry powder and cook for 1 minute, until fragrant. Add the coconut milk and bell peppers, turn the heat down to low, and simmer for about 10 minutes, until the chicken is cooked through.
2. Stir in the spinach and cook just until wilted. Season with salt and pepper before serving.

Nutritional Information (per serving): *Calories: 320; Protein: 24g; Carbohydrates: 10g; Fat: 20g; Fiber: 2g*

Coconut Curry Vegetable Stew

Servings: 4

2 tablespoons extra-virgin olive oil
1 medium onion, chopped
2 garlic cloves, minced
1 tablespoon grated fresh ginger
2 cups chopped mixed vegetables (such as carrots, peas, bell peppers)
1 (14-ounce) can coconut milk
2 cups vegetable broth
2 tablespoons yellow curry paste
Salt to taste

In a large saucepan, heat the olive oil over medium heat. Add the onion, garlic, and ginger and sauté until fragrant, 3 to 5 minutes. Stir in the mixed vegetables and cook for 5 minutes. Add the coconut milk, vegetable broth, curry paste, and salt. Turn the heat down to low and simmer for 15 to 20 minutes, until the vegetables are tender.

Nutritional Information (per serving): *Calories: 270; Protein: 4g; Carbohydrates: 18g; Fat: 20g; Fiber: 4g*

Curried Cauliflower and Lentils

Servings: 6

2 tablespoons extra-virgin olive oil
1 medium onion, chopped
2 garlic cloves, minced
1 head cauliflower, chopped into florets
1 cup red lentils, rinsed
2 tablespoons curry powder
4 cups vegetable broth
Salt and pepper to taste

In a large saucepan, heat the olive oil over medium heat. Add the onion and garlic and sauté until softened, 3 to 5 minutes. Add the cauliflower, red lentils, curry powder, and vegetable broth. Bring to a boil, then reduce the heat to low and simmer for 25 to 30 minutes, until the lentils are tender. Season with salt and pepper to taste.

Nutritional Information (per serving): *Calories: 190; Protein: 10g; Carbohydrates: 33g; Fat: 1g; Fiber: 10g*

Deviled Eggs

Servings: 6

12 hard-boiled eggs
2 tablespoons vegan mayo (I use vegan mayo for deviled eggs because it stands up in the heat better; egg-based mayo is food-safe for only up to 2 hours)
1 rounded tablespoon green sweet pickle relish
1 rounded tablespoon red pepper relish (I use Wickles brand)
1 rounded tablespoon yellow mustard
1 tablespoon Worcestershire sauce
1 tablespoon Frank's RedHot sauce or other hot sauce of choice
2 tablespoons freshly grated onion
1 garlic clove, minced
Salt and pepper to taste
12 slices jarred sweet or spicy Peppadew peppers, drained

Halve the eggs lengthwise and place the yolks in a medium bowl. Add the mayo, relishes, mustard, Worcestershire, hot sauce, onion, garlic, salt, and pepper to the bowl. Mash everything together well. Transfer the mixture to a zip-top plastic bag and seal. Snip off one bottom corner of the bag to make a pastry bag. Fill the egg white halves with the mixture. Top the stuffed eggs with the sliced peppers so the eggs look like devil eyes.

Nutritional Information (per serving): *Calories: 195; Protein: 12g; Carbohydrates: 6g; Fat: 13g; Fiber: 1g*

Dijon-Panko Chicken Tray Bake with Roasted Vegetables

Servings: 4

1 pound broccolini or green beans, trimmed
2 shallots, thinly sliced
2 tablespoons extra-virgin olive oil
Salt and pepper to taste
¼ cup Dijon mustard
Grated zest of 1 small lemon
4 tablespoons unsalted butter, softened
2 cups panko breadcrumbs
¼ cup chopped fresh flat-leaf parsley
2 tablespoons chopped fresh thyme
4 (6-ounce) boneless, skinless chicken breasts

1. Preheat the oven to 425°F (220°C). Line a rimmed baking sheet with parchment paper.
2. Bring a large pot of water to a boil. Fill a large bowl with cold water and ice. Add the broccolini or green beans to the boiling water and blanch for 2 minutes, then transfer to the ice bath until cool; drain well.
3. In a large bowl, toss the blanched vegetables with the shallots and olive oil. Season with salt and pepper and set aside.
4. In a small bowl, combine the Dijon, lemon zest, and softened butter. In a medium bowl, season the panko with the parsley and thyme.
5. Season the chicken with salt and pepper. Arrange the chicken on the prepared baking sheet, leaving space all around for the

veggies. Top each breast with a slather of mustard butter, then pack on the herbed panko.

6. Arrange the vegetable mixture around the chicken breasts. Roast for 22 to 25 minutes, until cooked through.

Nutritional Information (per serving): *Calories: 520; Protein: 45g; Carbohydrates: 30g; Fat: 27g; Fiber: 5g*

Grilled Mahi-Mahi with Mango Salsa

Servings: 4

Mango Salsa

1 ripe mango, peeled, pitted, and diced
½ medium red onion, finely chopped
1 jalapeño, seeded and diced
¼ cup chopped fresh cilantro
Juice of 1 lime

Mahi-Mahi

4 (6-ounce) mahi-mahi fillets
2 tablespoons extra-virgin olive oil
Juice of 1 lime
Salt and pepper to taste

1. Preheat the grill to medium-high heat.
2. In a medium bowl, combine all the salsa ingredients and toss well. Set aside.
3. Brush the mahi-mahi fillets with the olive oil and season with the lime juice, salt, and pepper. Grill the mahi-mahi for 5 to 6 minutes on each side, until the fish flakes easily with a fork.
4. Serve the mahi-mahi topped with the salsa.

Nutritional Information (per serving): *Calories: 350; Protein: 30g; Carbohydrates: 12g; Fat: 20g; Fiber: 2g*

Grilled Vegetable Skewers

Servings: 4

1 medium zucchini, sliced
1 bell pepper (any color), seeded and cut into pieces about the same size as the zucchini slices
1 medium red onion, cut into wedges
1 cup cherry tomatoes
2 tablespoons extra-virgin olive oil
1 teaspoon dried Italian seasoning
Salt and pepper to taste

1. Preheat the grill to medium heat.
2. In a large bowl, toss the zucchini, bell pepper, red onion, and cherry tomatoes with the olive oil, Italian seasoning, salt, and pepper.
3. Thread the vegetables onto skewers and grill, turning occasionally, for 10 to 15 minutes, until tender and lightly browned.

Nutritional Information (per serving): *Calories: 120; Protein: 3g; Carbohydrates: 9g; Fat: 8g; Fiber: 3g*

Gumbo Z'herbes

Servings: 8

For the gumbo

4 packed cups mustard greens, stems removed and leaves coarsely chopped
4 packed cups collard greens, stems removed and leaves coarsely chopped
4 packed cups turnip greens, stems removed and leaves coarsely chopped
4 packed cups beet greens, stems removed and leaves coarsely chopped
4 packed cups green or rainbow Swiss chard, stems removed and leaves coarsely chopped
2 packed cups spinach, coarsely chopped
2 packed cups romaine lettuce, coarsely chopped
1 packed cup chopped carrot fronds
1 packed cup chopped fresh flat-leaf parsley
1 red or green bell pepper, seeded and diced
1 medium yellow onion, chopped
2 medium carrots, finely chopped
2 medium celery ribs with leafy tops, finely chopped
1 cilantro sprig, 1 thyme sprig, and 1 bay leaf tied together into a bundle
2 quarts vegetable or chicken broth
2 quarts water

To serve

1 pound andouille sausage links, sliced into ½-inch rounds
3 tablespoons vegetable oil
3 tablespoons all-purpose flour
1½ teaspoons filé powder (gumbo filé)
Salt and pepper to taste
6 cups cooked basmati rice
Thinly sliced scallions, for garnish
Hot sauce, for serving

1. In a large pot, combine all the gumbo ingredients and bring to a boil. Reduce the heat to a simmer and cook for 1 hour.
2. When the gumbo is nearly done, cook the sausage in a large skillet over medium heat until browned, about 10 minutes, then transfer to paper towels to drain.
3. Add the vegetable oil and flour to the drippings left in the pan and cook, stirring constantly, until golden, about 5 minutes, then whisk in the filé powder. Stir this roux and the sausage into the pot of gumbo. Season with salt and pepper.
4. Serve the gumbo topped with ice-cream scoopfuls of rice and a sprinkle of scallions, with hot sauce to taste.

Nutritional Information (per serving): *Calories: 420; Protein: 18g; Carbohydrates: 40g; Fat: 20g; Fiber: 8g*

Lemon-Garlic Baked Salmon

Servings: 4

3 tablespoons extra-virgin olive oil
Juice of 1 lemon
4 garlic cloves, minced
Salt and pepper to taste
4 (6-ounce) salmon fillets
Chopped fresh flat-leaf parsley, for garnish

1. Preheat the oven to 400°F (200°C). Line a rimmed baking sheet with parchment paper.
2. In a small bowl, mix the olive oil, lemon juice, garlic, salt, and pepper.
3. Place the salmon fillets on the prepared baking sheet. Brush the fillets with the lemon-garlic mixture. Bake for 12 to 15 minutes, until the salmon flakes easily with a fork.
4. Garnish with parsley before serving.

Nutritional Information (per serving): *Calories: 320; Protein: 34g; Carbohydrates: 0g; Fat: 20g; Fiber: 0g*

Lemon-Garlic Shrimp with Quinoa

Servings: 4

2 tablespoons extra-virgin olive oil
2 garlic cloves, minced
1 pound large shrimp, peeled and deveined, tails removed
Juice of 1 lemon
Salt and pepper to taste
2 cups cooked quinoa
Chopped fresh flat-leaf parsley, for garnish

1. In a large skillet, heat the olive oil over medium heat. Add the garlic and sauté for 1 minute. Add the shrimp, lemon juice, salt, and pepper and cook, stirring occasionally, until the shrimp are pink, 4 to 5 minutes.
2. Serve the shrimp over the quinoa, garnished with parsley.

Nutritional Information (per serving): *Calories: 280; Protein: 26g; Carbohydrates: 24g; Fat: 10g; Fiber: 2g*

Lemon-Herb Grilled Chicken

Servings: 4

2 tablespoons extra-virgin olive oil
Grated zest and juice of 1 lemon
3 garlic cloves, minced
1 teaspoon dried oregano
1 teaspoon dried thyme
Salt and pepper to taste
4 (6-ounce) boneless, skinless chicken breasts

1. In a small bowl, whisk together the olive oil, lemon zest and juice, garlic, oregano, thyme, salt, and pepper.
2. Place the chicken breasts in a resealable plastic bag or shallow dish and pour the marinade over them. Seal the bag (or cover the dish) and marinate in the refrigerator for at least 30 minutes, or preferably up to 3 hours.
3. Preheat the grill to medium-high heat. Grill the chicken for 6 to 7 minutes on each side, until cooked through.

Nutritional Information (per serving): *Calories: 220; Protein: 28g; Carbohydrates: 2g; Fat: 11g; Fiber: 0g*

Lentil and Spinach Soup

Servings: 6

2 tablespoons extra-virgin olive oil
1 medium onion, chopped
2 garlic cloves, minced
2 medium carrots, diced
1 cup green lentils, rinsed
6 cups vegetable broth
1 teaspoon dried thyme
2 cups chopped fresh spinach
Salt and pepper to taste

In a large pot, heat the olive oil over medium heat. Add the onion and garlic and sauté until translucent, 3 to 5 minutes. Add the carrots and green lentils and cook, stirring, for 2 minutes. Pour in the vegetable broth and thyme and bring to a boil. Reduce the heat and simmer for 30 minutes. Stir in the spinach and cook just until wilted. Season with salt and pepper to taste.

Nutritional Information (per serving): *Calories: 210; Protein: 14g; Carbohydrates: 34g; Fat: 4g; Fiber: 12g*

Lentil Bolognese with Whole Wheat Spaghetti

Servings: 4

2 tablespoons extra-virgin olive oil
1 medium onion, chopped
2 medium carrots, diced
2 medium celery ribs, diced
3 garlic cloves, minced
½ cup green or brown lentils, rinsed
1 (14-ounce) can crushed tomatoes
1 teaspoon dried oregano
Salt and pepper to taste
4 ounces dried whole wheat spaghetti

1. In a large pot, heat the olive oil over medium heat. Add the onion, carrots, and celery and sauté for about 5 minutes, until softened. Add the garlic, lentils, crushed tomatoes, oregano, salt, and pepper. Bring to a boil, then reduce the heat and simmer for 25 to 30 minutes, until the lentils are tender.
2. Meanwhile, cook the spaghetti according to the package instructions; drain.
3. Serve the lentil Bolognese over the spaghetti.

Nutritional Information (per serving): *Calories: 350; Protein: 12g; Carbohydrates: 40g; Fat: 16g; Fiber: 10g*

Mediterranean Chickpea Salad

Servings: 4

1 (15-ounce) can chickpeas, rinsed and drained
1 cup cherry tomatoes, halved
1 cucumber, diced
½ medium red onion, chopped
¼ cup chopped fresh flat-leaf parsley
3 tablespoons extra-virgin olive oil
2 tablespoons lemon juice
Salt and pepper to taste

1. In a large bowl, combine the chickpeas, cherry tomatoes, cucumber, red onion, and parsley.
2. In a small bowl, whisk together the olive oil, lemon juice, salt, and pepper.
3. Pour the dressing over the salad and toss gently.

Nutritional Information (per serving): *Calories: 230; Protein: 5g; Carbohydrates: 22g; Fat: 12g; Fiber: 6g*

Mediterranean Cod with Tomatoes and Olives

Servings: 4

1 (14-ounce) can diced tomatoes
½ cup kalamata olives, pitted and sliced
2 tablespoons capers, rinsed
2 garlic cloves, minced
2 tablespoons extra-virgin olive oil
1 teaspoon dried oregano
Salt and pepper to taste
4 (6-ounce) cod fillets
Chopped fresh basil, for garnish

1. Preheat the oven to 375°F (190°C).
2. In a large baking dish, combine the diced tomatoes with their juice, olives, capers, garlic, olive oil, oregano, salt, and pepper. Place the cod fillets on top of the tomato mixture. Bake for 20 to 25 minutes, or until the fish is opaque and flakes easily with a fork. Garnish with basil before serving.

Nutritional Information (per serving): *Calories: 290; Protein: 34g; Carbohydrates: 10g; Fat: 12g; Fiber: 2g*

Mediterranean Lentil Soup

Servings: 6

2 tablespoons extra-virgin olive oil
1 medium onion, chopped
2 medium carrots, diced
2 medium celery ribs, diced
2 garlic cloves, minced
1 cup green or brown lentils, rinsed
4 cups vegetable broth
1 (14-ounce) can diced tomatoes
2 teaspoons ground cumin
Salt and pepper to taste

In a large pot, heat the olive oil over medium heat. Add the onion, carrots, and celery and sauté until softened, 10 to 12 minutes. Add the garlic and cook for another minute. Stir in the lentils, vegetable broth, tomatoes with their juice, cumin, salt, and pepper. Bring to a boil, then reduce the heat and simmer for 30 to 40 minutes, until the lentils are tender.

Nutritional Information (per serving): *Calories: 210; Protein: 12g; Carbohydrates: 36g; Fat: 1g; Fiber: 12g*

Mediterranean Orzo Salad

Servings: 4

1 cup whole wheat orzo
1 (15-ounce) can chickpeas, rinsed and drained
1 cup cherry tomatoes, halved
1 cucumber, diced
¼ cup red onion, finely chopped
¼ cup crumbled feta cheese (optional)
2 tablespoons extra-virgin olive oil
2 tablespoons red wine vinegar
1 teaspoon dried oregano
Salt and pepper to taste

1. Cook the orzo according to the package instructions. Drain and rinse under cold water.
2. In a large bowl, combine the cooked orzo, chickpeas, cherry tomatoes, cucumber, red onion, and feta (if using).
3. In a small bowl, whisk together the olive oil, vinegar, oregano, salt, and pepper.
4. Drizzle the dressing over the salad and toss to combine.

Nutritional Information (per serving): *Calories: 320; Protein: 10g; Carbohydrates: 40g; Fat: 13g; Fiber: 8g*

Mystic, Connecticut–Style Portuguese Stew

Servings: 6

2 tablespoons extra-virgin olive oil
1 pound chourico, chorizo, or smoked linguica (I like the hot chourico from Gaspar's), casings removed and cut into bite-size pieces
1 pound baby white potatoes, quartered
1 medium onion, chopped
2 celery ribs with leafy tops, chopped
6 garlic cloves, chopped
1 large bay leaf
1 hot red chile pepper, chopped
1 red bell pepper, chopped
Salt and pepper to taste
1 (14-ounce) can diced tomatoes
3 cups chicken broth
1 pound boneless, skinless chicken thighs, cut into bite-size pieces, or 1 pound large shrimp, peeled, deveined, and butterflied
½ cup chopped fresh flat-leaf parsley

Heat the olive oil in a large, deep skillet or pot over medium heat. Add the sausage and cook for a minute or two to let some of the fat render out. Add the baby white potatoes, onion, celery, garlic, bay leaf, and chopped peppers and season with salt and pepper. Cover the pan and let the vegetables sweat for 10 to 12 minutes. Add the tomatoes with their juice and chicken broth and continue to simmer, covered, for another 5 minutes. Add the chicken and poach until the chicken is cooked through and the potatoes are fork-tender, 10 to 12 minutes. Add the parsley and serve.

Nutritional Information (per serving): *Calories: 405; Protein: 25g; Carbohydrates: 21g; Fat: 24g; Fiber: 4g*

Oysters and Mignonette

Servings: 6

1 shallot, finely chopped
1 teaspoon salt
½ cup red wine vinegar, white wine vinegar, or champagne vinegar
2 teaspoons pepper
1 lemon, seeded and cut into wedges
24 Kumamoto or Pink Moon oysters, scrubbed and shucked

1. In a small bowl, season the shallot with the salt and let sweat for a few minutes, then add the vinegar and pepper.
2. To serve, fill a serving bowl with ice and arrange the lemon wedges and oysters on top. Serve with the mignonette sauce.

Nutritional Information (per serving): *Calories: 70; Protein: 7g; Carbohydrates: 3g; Fat: 2g; Fiber: 0g*

Pasta con le Sarde

Servings: 6

For the dried fruit

½ cup dry vermouth, dry white wine, or water

1 fat pinch saffron (20 to 24 threads)

¼ cup golden raisins, chopped, or currants

For the pasta

1 pound dried bucatini (hollow spaghetti) or chitarra (square-cut spaghetti)

¼ cup extra-virgin olive oil

4 flat anchovy fillets in oil, drained

1 teaspoon fennel seeds

1 fennel bulb, quartered, cored, and finely chopped, fronds chopped for garnish

1 medium yellow onion, finely chopped

Salt and black pepper to taste

1 fat pinch red pepper flakes

4 garlic cloves, finely chopped

1 pound fresh sardine fillets, boned and cut into bite-size pieces, or 2 (3.75-ounce) cans sardine fillets, drained and broken up with a fork

¼ cup pine nuts, toasted

2 tablespoons chopped fresh flat-leaf parsley

1. In a small saucepan, bring the dry vermouth and saffron to a low boil over medium-low heat. Remove from the heat, add the golden raisins, and let the fruit bloom for 10 to 15 minutes.
2. Meanwhile, bring a large pot of salted water to a boil. Add the pasta and cook for 1 minute less than the package instructions as it will continue to cook in the sauce. Scoop out ½ cup of the pasta cooking water, then drain the pasta.

3. Heat the olive oil in a large skillet over medium heat. Add the anchovies and let them melt into the oil, breaking them up with a wooden spoon or paddle. Stir in the fennel seeds, chopped fennel bulb, and yellow onion and season with salt, black pepper, and red pepper flakes. Cook, stirring, for 2 to 3 minutes. Add the garlic and stir, then add the golden raisins and their soaking liquid. Add the sardines and cook for 2 minutes more.
4. Add the pasta and reserved ½ cup pasta cooking water to the sauce and mix well.
5. Transfer the pasta to a warm serving bowl or serve from the skillet, topped with the pine nuts, parsley, and fennel fronds.

Nutritional Information (per serving): *Calories: 70; Protein: 8g; Carbohydrates: 3g; Fat: 2g; Fiber: 1g*

Pasta Primavera with Whole Wheat Penne

Servings: 4

8 ounces dried whole wheat penne
2 tablespoons extra-virgin olive oil
3 garlic cloves, minced
2 cups chopped mixed vegetables (such as bell peppers, broccoli, carrots, zucchini)
Salt and pepper to taste
¼ cup grated Parmesan cheese (optional)
Chopped fresh basil, for garnish

1. Cook the penne according to the package instructions. Drain.
2. Meanwhile, in a large skillet, heat the olive oil over medium heat. Add the garlic and sauté for 1 minute. Add the mixed vegetables and cook for 5 to 7 minutes, until tender-crisp.
3. Add the cooked penne to the skillet and toss to combine. Season with salt and pepper.
4. Serve topped with Parmesan cheese (if using) and basil.

Nutritional Information (per serving): *Calories: 280; Protein: 10g; Carbohydrates: 45g; Fat: 9g; Fiber: 7g*

Portuguese Chicken

Servings: 4

8 (6-ounce) bone-in, skin-on chicken thighs or 4 large whole chicken legs (drums attached to thighs)
1 tablespoon dried piri-piri (ground Portuguese chiles) or ground ancho chiles
1 tablespoon smoked sweet paprika (pimentón)
1 handful fresh cilantro, finely chopped
Salt and pepper to taste
Extra-virgin olive oil spray
1 pound hot Portuguese chourico (such as Gaspar's) or meaty Spanish chorizo, casings removed and sliced on a bias ½- to ¾-inch thick
1 medium carrot, finely chopped
1 large celery rib with leafy tops, finely chopped
1 medium yellow onion, finely chopped
1 small red bell pepper, finely chopped
1 Fresno or other mild chile pepper, finely chopped
4 garlic cloves, chopped
1 lemon, halved
2 tablespoons red vinegar
3 tablespoons tomato paste
1½ cups chicken broth

1. Preheat the oven to 425°F (220°C).
2. Season the chicken with the ground chiles, paprika, cilantro, salt, and pepper.
3. Heat a large cast-iron skillet over medium-high heat and spray with olive oil. Add the chicken, skin side down, and brown for 5 minutes, then turn and brown the other side for 3 to 4 minutes more. Transfer to a platter.

4. Lower the heat to medium. Add the sausage and cook for just a minute or so on each side to render the fat, then transfer to the platter with the chicken.
5. Add the carrot, celery, yellow onion, chopped peppers, garlic, and lemon halves, cut sides down. Season with salt and pepper. Once the lemon has browned a bit, stir in the red vinegar, tomato paste, and chicken broth.
6. Return the chicken and sausage to the pan and cook for 5 to 7 minutes, until the chicken is cooked through.

Nutritional Information (per serving): *Calories: 540; Protein: 28g; Carbohydrates: 52g; Fat: 23g; Fiber: 5g*

Quinoa and Black Bean Salad

Servings: 4

1 cup cooked quinoa
1 (15-ounce) can black beans, rinsed and drained
1 cup diced red and/or yellow bell peppers
1 cup fresh or thawed frozen corn
1 medium avocado, peeled, pitted, and diced
2 tablespoons lime juice
2 tablespoons extra-virgin olive oil
1 teaspoon ground cumin
Salt and pepper to taste

1. In a large bowl, combine the quinoa, black beans, bell peppers, corn, and avocado.
2. In a small bowl, whisk together the lime juice, olive oil, cumin, salt, and pepper.
3. Pour the dressing over the salad and toss gently. Serve chilled.

Nutritional Information (per serving): *Calories: 320; Protein: 12g; Carbohydrates: 42g; Fat: 14g; Fiber: 12g*

Quinoa and Roasted Vegetable Bowl

Servings: 4

1 medium zucchini, diced
1 bell pepper, diced
1 medium red onion, diced
2 tablespoons extra-virgin olive oil
Salt and pepper to taste
1 cup cooked quinoa
1 tablespoon balsamic vinegar

1. Preheat the oven to 425°F (220°C).
2. On a rimmed baking sheet, toss the zucchini, bell pepper, and red onion with the olive oil, salt, and pepper. Spread out in a single layer and roast for 20 to 25 minutes, until lightly browned.
3. Transfer the roasted vegetables to a large bowl, add the quinoa and balsamic vinegar, and toss well.

Nutritional Information (per serving): *Calories: 260; Protein: 8g; Carbohydrates: 40g; Fat: 8g; Fiber: 7g*

Roasted Beet and Goat Cheese Salad

Servings: 4

4 cups mixed greens
2 medium beets, roasted and sliced
¼ cup crumbled goat cheese
¼ cup walnuts, toasted
2 tablespoons balsamic vinaigrette
Salt and pepper to taste

In a large bowl, combine the mixed greens, beets, goat cheese, and walnuts. Drizzle with the balsamic vinaigrette and season with salt and pepper. Toss gently to combine.

Nutritional Information (per serving): *Calories: 210; Protein: 6g; Carbohydrates: 15g; Fat: 15g; Fiber: 4g*

Roasted Sweet Potato and Chickpea Bowl

Servings: 4

1 medium sweet potato, peeled and cubed
1 (15-ounce) can chickpeas, rinsed and drained
2 tablespoons extra-virgin olive oil
1 teaspoon paprika
1 teaspoon garlic powder
Salt and pepper to taste
2 cups chopped kale

1. Preheat the oven to 400°F (200°C).
2. On a rimmed baking sheet, toss the sweet potato and chickpeas with the olive oil, paprika, garlic powder, salt, and pepper. Spread out in a single layer and roast for 25 to 30 minutes, until golden.
3. In a serving bowl, add the kale, then the roasted sweet potato and chickpeas.

Nutritional Information (per serving): *Calories: 290; Protein: 10g; Carbohydrates: 46g; Fat: 10g; Fiber: 11g*

Spicy Hummus with Veggies

Servings: 4

1 (15-ounce) can chickpeas, rinsed and drained
2 tablespoons tahini
2 tablespoons extra-virgin olive oil
1 garlic clove, crushed
1 teaspoon ground cumin
1 teaspoon cayenne pepper, or to taste
Salt to taste
Raw cut-up veggies (such as carrots, cucumbers, bell peppers), for dipping

1. In a food processor, blend the chickpeas, tahini, olive oil, garlic, cumin, cayenne, and salt until smooth.
2. Serve with raw vegetables for dipping.

Nutritional Information (per serving): *Calories: 180; Protein: 6g; Carbohydrates: 22g; Fat: 8g; Fiber: 6g*

Spicy Shrimp and Quinoa Bowl

Servings: 4

1 pound large shrimp, peeled and deveined, tails removed
4 tablespoons extra-virgin olive oil, divided
1 teaspoon chili powder
½ teaspoon ground cumin
½ teaspoon garlic powder
Salt and pepper to taste
1 cup cooked quinoa
1 cup mixed greens
1 medium avocado, peeled, pitted, and sliced

1. In a bowl, toss the shrimp with 2 tablespoons of the olive oil, the chili powder, cumin, garlic powder, salt, and pepper.
2. Heat the remaining 2 tablespoons olive oil in a large skillet over medium-high heat. Add the shrimp and cook for 2 to 3 minutes on each side, until pink and opaque.
3. Divide the quinoa into bowls and top with the shrimp, mixed greens, and avocado slices.

***Nutritional Information (per serving):** Calories: 405; Protein: 28g; Carbohydrates: 26g; Fat: 22g; Fiber: 6g*

Spinach and Feta Stuffed Chicken Breasts

Servings: 4

1 cup chopped fresh spinach
½ cup crumbled feta cheese
2 tablespoons chopped sun-dried tomatoes
4 (6-ounce) boneless, skinless chicken breasts
1 tablespoon extra-virgin olive oil
1 teaspoon garlic powder
Salt and pepper to taste

1. Preheat the oven to 375°F (190°C).
2. In a medium bowl, combine the spinach, feta, and sun-dried tomatoes and mix well.
3. Using a sharp knife, create a pocket by slicing horizontally into the thickest part of each chicken breast. Stuff each breast with the spinach mixture. Rub the olive oil over the chicken breasts and season with the garlic powder, salt, and pepper.
4. Place the stuffed chicken breasts in a baking dish and bake for 25 to 30 minutes, until the chicken is cooked through.

Nutritional Information (per serving): *Calories: 290; Protein: 30g; Carbohydrates: 3g; Fat: 17g; Fiber: 1g*

Spinach and Feta Stuffed Peppers

Servings: 4

2 cups cooked brown rice
1 cup chopped fresh spinach
½ cup crumbled feta cheese
1 teaspoon extra-virgin olive oil
1 teaspoon dried oregano
Salt and pepper to taste
4 red or yellow bell peppers, halved lengthwise and seeded

1. Preheat the oven to 375°F (190°C).
2. In a large bowl, combine the brown rice, spinach, feta, olive oil, oregano, salt, and pepper and mix well. Stuff the mixture into the pepper halves.
3. Place the stuffed peppers in a baking dish and cover with aluminum foil. Bake for 25 minutes.

Nutritional Information (per serving): *Calories: 230; Protein: 8g; Carbohydrates: 36g; Fat: 7g; Fiber: 5g*

Spinach and Mushroom Quesadilla

Servings: 2

1 tablespoon extra-virgin olive oil
1 cup sliced mushrooms
1 cup chopped fresh spinach
2 whole-grain tortillas
½ cup shredded cheddar or mozzarella cheese

1. In a large skillet, heat the olive oil over medium heat. Add the mushrooms and sauté until soft, about 15 minutes. Add the spinach and cook just until wilted. Transfer the mushroom and spinach mixture to a bowl.
2. Place one tortilla in the skillet, add the mushroom-spinach mixture in an even layer, sprinkle the cheese evenly over the vegetables, and top with the second tortilla. Cook over medium heat until golden, 1 to 2 minutes, then carefully flip and cook on the other side for another 1 minute. Slice and serve.

Nutritional Information (per serving): *Calories: 320; Protein: 14g; Carbohydrates: 34g; Fat: 14g; Fiber: 5g*

Stuffed Acorn Squash

Servings: 4

2 medium acorn squashes
2 tablespoons extra-virgin olive oil
Salt and pepper to taste
1 cup cooked quinoa or brown rice
1 (15-ounce) can black beans, rinsed and drained
1 cup fresh, thawed frozen, or drained canned corn
1 bell pepper (any color), seeded and diced
¼ cup finely chopped red onion
¼ cup chopped fresh cilantro (optional)
Juice of 1 lime, plus lime wedges for serving (optional)
1 teaspoon ground cumin
1 teaspoon chili powder
½ cup shredded cheddar or mozzarella cheese (optional)

1. Preheat the oven to 400°F (200°C).
2. Carefully slice the acorn squashes in half from stem to bottom. Remove the seeds and stringy insides using a spoon. Place the squash halves cut side up on a rimmed baking sheet. Drizzle with the olive oil and season with salt and pepper. Flip the squash halves cut side down and roast for 25 to 30 minutes, until the flesh is tender and easily pierced with a fork.
3. While the squash is roasting, in a large bowl, combine the quinoa, black beans, corn, bell pepper, red onion, cilantro (if using), lime juice, cumin, chili powder, salt, and pepper. Mix well to combine all the ingredients.
4. Once the squash is done roasting, remove it from the oven and carefully flip each half over so the cut side is facing up. Spoon the

filling mixture into each acorn squash half, packing it in gently. If using cheese, sprinkle it on top of the filling.

5. Return the stuffed squash to the oven and bake for an additional 10 to 15 minutes, until everything is heated through and the cheese is melted (if using).
6. Let cool slightly. Garnish with additional cilantro and serve with lime wedges, if desired.

Nutritional Information (per serving): *Calories: 360; Protein: 14g; Carbohydrates: 56g; Fat: 10g; Fiber: 12g*

Thai Red Curry with Shrimp

Servings: 6

Thai Yogurt Sauce

1 cup plain Greek yogurt

¼ cup natural peanut butter

Juice of 1 small lime

2 tablespoons light soy sauce

1 garlic clove, minced

½-inch piece fresh ginger, peeled and grated

Shrimp Curry

2 tablespoons ghee, coconut oil, or avocado oil

1 medium red onion, chopped

1 large red bell pepper, seeded and chopped

4 hot Thai chiles, seeded and finely chopped

4 garlic cloves, minced

1-inch piece fresh ginger, peeled and grated

¼ cup red curry paste

2 teaspoons cornstarch

2 (14-ounce) cans coconut milk

1 pound large shrimp, peeled, deveined, and butterflied

1 tablespoon chopped fresh basil

Grated zest and juice of 1 lime

Flatbreads, for serving (optional)

4 cups cooked jasmine or basmati rice

Sriracha, for serving (optional)

1. Combine all the yogurt sauce ingredients in a bowl and mix well. Cover and chill until ready to serve.

2. Heat the ghee or oil in a large skillet over medium-high heat. Add the red onion, red bell pepper, and hot chiles and cook, stirring, for a couple of minutes, then add the garlic, ginger, and curry paste and cook for another 2 or 3 minutes.
3. In a small bowl, make a slurry by whisking together the cornstarch and a splash of warm water.
4. Add the coconut milk to the skillet, then stir in the slurry to thicken. When the sauce bubbles, add the shrimp and cook until opaque and firm, 3 to 5 minutes. Remove from the heat. Add the basil and let it wilt, then stir in the lime zest and juice.
5. Let the mixture sit for 5 minutes.
6. Meanwhile, if serving with flatbreads, heat a nonstick griddle pan over medium heat, add a little water, and char the flatbreads on each side.
7. Serve the curry with the rice and flatbreads (if using). Add a dollop of yogurt sauce on top and a dash of sriracha, if you like.

Nutritional Information (per serving): *Calories: 475; Protein: 25g; Carbohydrates: 45g; Fat: 21g; Fiber: 5g*

Tomato Basil Soup

Servings: 4

1 tablespoon extra-virgin olive oil

1 medium onion, chopped

2 garlic cloves, minced

1 (28-ounce) can crushed tomatoes

2 cups vegetable broth

Salt and pepper to taste

¼ cup chopped fresh basil

In a medium saucepan, heat the olive oil over medium heat. Add the onion and garlic and sauté until softened, about 5 minutes. Add the crushed tomatoes with their liquid, vegetable broth, salt, and pepper. Bring to a boil, then reduce the heat and simmer for 20 minutes. Stir in the basil before serving.

Nutritional Information (per serving): *Calories: 130; Protein: 4g; Carbohydrates: 20g; Fat: 4g; Fiber: 4g*

Tuna Salad with Avocado and Chickpeas

Servings: 4

3 (5-ounce) cans tuna in water, drained
1 medium avocado, peeled, pitted, and diced
1 cup rinsed and drained canned chickpeas
¼ cup finely chopped red onion
¼ cup chopped fresh cilantro
Juice of 1 lime
Salt and pepper to taste
Whole-grain bread, lettuce, or mixed greens, for serving

In a large bowl, combine the tuna, avocado, chickpeas, red onion, and cilantro. Drizzle with the lime juice and season with salt and pepper. Gently mix to combine without mashing the avocado. Serve as a sandwich, in lettuce wraps, or on top of a salad.

Nutritional Information (per serving): *Calories: 310; Protein: 22g; Carbohydrates: 24g; Fat: 15g; Fiber: 8g*

Vegetable Stir-Fry with Tofu

Servings: 4

1 tablespoon toasted sesame oil
2 garlic cloves, minced
1 teaspoon grated fresh ginger
1 (14-ounce) block firm tofu, drained and cubed
2 cups chopped mixed vegetables (such as broccoli, bell peppers, carrots)
2 tablespoons soy sauce or tamari

Heat the sesame oil in a large skillet over medium heat. Add the garlic and ginger and sauté for 1 minute. Add the tofu and cook until golden on all sides, 10 to 15 minutes. Add the mixed vegetables and soy sauce and stir-fry for 5 to 7 minutes, until crisp-tender and lightly browned.

Nutritional Information (per serving): *Calories: 210; Protein: 12g; Carbohydrates: 16g; Fat: 12g; Fiber: 4g*

Whole Wheat Pasta with Spinach and Chickpeas

Servings: 4

8 ounces dried whole wheat pasta
2 tablespoons extra-virgin olive oil
2 garlic cloves, minced
1 (15-ounce) can chickpeas, rinsed and drained
3 cups chopped fresh spinach
Juice of 1 lemon
Salt and pepper to taste
¼ cup grated Parmesan cheese (optional)

1. Cook the pasta according to the package instructions. Reserve ½ cup of the pasta cooking water, then drain.
2. In a large skillet, heat the olive oil over medium heat. Add the garlic and sauté for 1 minute. Stir in the chickpeas and spinach and cook just until the spinach is wilted.
3. Add the cooked pasta and lemon juice and toss to combine, adding some of the reserved pasta cooking water as needed to reach the desired consistency.
4. Season with salt and pepper and top with Parmesan cheese, if desired.

Nutritional Information (per serving): *Calories: 320; Protein: 12g; Carbohydrates: 50g; Fat: 10g; Fiber: 8g*

Zucchini Noodles with Pesto and Cherry Tomatoes

Servings: 4

2 tablespoons extra-virgin olive oil
1 cup cherry tomatoes, halved
4 medium zucchini, spiralized into noodles
¼ cup basil pesto
Salt and pepper to taste
Fresh basil, for garnish

In a large skillet, heat the olive oil over medium heat. Add the cherry tomatoes and sauté for about 5 minutes, until they begin to soften. Add the zucchini noodles and cook for 2 to 3 minutes, just until heated through. Stir in the pesto and toss until well combined. Season with salt and pepper. Serve immediately, garnished with fresh basil.

Nutritional Information (per serving): *Calories: 180; Protein: 4g; Carbohydrates: 14g; Fat: 14g; Fiber: 3g*

Appendix II: Snack Well, Snack Smart

Snacking often gets a bad reputation, especially when associated with mindless eating or ultra-processed convenience foods. But when done intentionally and nutritionally, snacking can be a powerful ally during the menopausal transition. As hormone levels fluctuate, women often experience increased hunger, shifts in blood sugar, disrupted sleep, and mood swings—conditions that can be soothed and stabilized with the right nourishment, timed strategically throughout the day.

Menopause-friendly snacking isn't about restriction or complicated meal prep. It's about adding value—foods that nourish your body, support your changing metabolism, and keep your energy steady without the crash. A well-chosen snack can reduce cravings, support hormone balance, improve bone and brain health, and even help relieve hot flashes and mood dips.

What makes this approach to combining specific foods even more empowering is its simplicity and affordability. These snacks are built around real, whole ingredients that are easy to find in any grocery store. Many require minimal prep, can be made in batches ahead of time, and are portable for busy days. Whether you're between meetings, running errands, or relaxing at home, these choices fit naturally into any routine. They're a practical, delicious way to move away from processed, packaged foods loaded with added sugar, sodium, and preservatives—ingredients that can worsen inflammation, disrupt hormones, and contribute to weight gain during midlife. More than just fillers between meals, these snacks are functional, flavorful building blocks of a supportive menopausal lifestyle.

The following snack list is curated with these principles in mind: balance, benefit, and simplicity. Let's take a look at seventy-five menopause-friendly snacks designed to support your body, your hormones, and your life—one bite at a time.

Almond Butter on Rice Cakes (120 cal)
1 rice cake + 1 tablespoon almond butter

Apple Slices with Tahini (120 cal)
1 small apple + 1 tablespoon tahini

Avocado Deviled Eggs (180 cal)
2 halves of a hard-boiled egg filled with mashed avocado

Avocado on Whole-Grain Crackers (150 cal)
3 crackers + ¼ avocado, mashed

Baked Plantain Chips (180 cal)
½ cup

Berry Ice Cubes in Sparkling Water (60 cal)
1 glass with 4 or 5 berry ice cubes

Blueberry Protein Shake (200 cal)
1 cup unsweetened almond milk + 20 grams protein powder + ½ cup blueberries + ½ small banana; ice chips optional to make it cold, or use frozen blueberries

Blueberry Walnut Mix (150 cal)
½ cup fresh blueberries + 1 tablespoon chopped walnuts

Butternut Squash Bites (100 cal)
½ cup butternut squash, cubed and roasted in 1 tablespoon olive oil

Carrot Sticks with Almond Dip (150 cal)
1 cup carrot sticks + 2 tablespoons dip

Celery with Sunflower Seed Butter (150 cal)
3 celery ribs + 2 tablespoons sunflower seed butter

Cherry Tomatoes with Feta Crumbles (150 cal)
1 cup cherry tomatoes + 1 tablespoon feta cheese

Chia and Almond Milk Mini Shake (150 cal)
1 cup almond milk + 2 tablespoons chia seeds + 1 small frozen banana, sliced

Chia Yogurt Bowl with Almond Butter (150 cal)
½ cup yogurt + 1 tablespoon almond butter + 1 tablespoon chia seeds

Chilled Herbal Hibiscus Tea with Orange Slices (30 cal)
12 ounces tea + 2 whole orange slices

Cinnamon Baked Apple Slices (80 cal)
1 medium apple, cored, sliced, sprinkled with cinnamon, and baked

Coconut Yogurt with Berries and Ground Hemp (150 cal)
¾ cup coconut milk yogurt + ¼ cup mixed fresh berries + 1 teaspoon hemp

Coconut Yogurt with Lime Zest (120 cal)
¾ cup coconut milk yogurt + zest of 1 lime

Cottage Cheese with Flaxseeds (180 cal)
½ cup cottage cheese + 1 teaspoon flaxseeds

Cottage Cheese with Pineapple Chunks (180 cal)
½ cup cottage cheese + ¼ cup pineapple chunks

Cucumber Slices with Greek Tzatziki (70 cal)
1 cup cucumber slices + 2 tablespoons tzatziki

Dark Chocolate–Covered Almonds (150 cal)
10 almonds

Dark Chocolate–Covered Banana Slices (150 cal)
½ medium banana, sliced, dipped in chocolate, and frozen

Edamame with Sea Salt (180 cal)
1 cup steamed

Frozen Grapes and Dark Chocolate Chips (150 cal)
½ cup grapes + 1 tablespoon chocolate chips

Frozen Kiwi Slices (50 cal)
1 kiwi, peeled, sliced, and frozen

Frozen Mango Cubes (150 cal)
½ cup frozen chunks

Golden Beet Chips (150 cal)
½ cup

Greek Yogurt and Walnuts (150 cal)
¾ cup yogurt + 1 tablespoon walnuts

Guacamole and Jicama Sticks (180 cal)
¼ cup guacamole + 1 cup jicama sticks

Hard-Boiled Egg and Avocado Slices (180 cal)
1 egg + ¼ avocado

Hard-Boiled Egg with Olive Tapenade (180 cal)
1 egg + 1 tablespoon tapenade

Hard-Boiled Eggs with Pesto Dip (230 cal)
2 eggs + 1 tablespoon pesto

Herbal Cucumber Bites (50 cal)
6 cucumber slices + fresh herbs

Hummus and Bell Pepper Strips (150 cal)
¼ cup hummus + 1 cup peppers

Lentil Crackers with Hummus (180 cal)
8 crackers + 2 tablespoons hummus

Lentil Salad Cup (180 cal)
½ cup cooked lentils + ¼ cup each of diced tomatoes and cucumbers

Mashed Banana with Hemp and Cinnamon (150 cal)
½ medium banana + 1 teaspoon hemp + cinnamon

Mashed Sweet Potato with Cinnamon (180 cal)
1 cup sweet potato + cinnamon

Melon and Pumpkin Seed Bowl (150 cal)
½ cup melon + 1 tablespoon pumpkin seeds

Mini Turkey Roll-Ups with Spinach (150 cal)
Spinach + 2 slices fresh deli turkey

Mozzarella and Tomato Skewers (150 cal)
3 skewers: 3 cherry tomatoes and 2 small cubes mozzarella each

Oat Milk Chai Latte (150 cal)
1 cup

Pear Slices and Almond Butter (150 cal)
½ pear + 1 tablespoon almond butter

Pear Slices with Goat Cheese Crumbles (150 cal)
½ pear + 1 tablespoon goat cheese

Pineapple and Mint Salad (85 cal)
½ cup fresh pineapple chunks + fresh mint

Pistachio and Dried Cherry Mix (150 cal)
2 tablespoons each

Pumpkin Seed and Dried Cranberry Mix (150 cal)
2 tablespoons pumpkin seeds + 1 tablespoon dried cranberries

Pumpkin Yogurt Bowl (150 cal)
½ cup yogurt + ¼ cup pumpkin puree

Red Bell Pepper Hummus Cups (150 cal)
2 pepper halves + 2 tablespoons hummus

Red Grapes and Goat Cheese Skewers (150 cal)
1 skewer: 5 grapes + 1 ounce cheese, cubed

Ricotta on Rice Cake with Cinnamon (150 cal)
1 rice cake + ¼ cup ricotta + cinnamon

Roasted Broccoli Florets (100 cal)
2 cups

Roasted Carrots with Tahini Drizzle (150 cal)
½ cup carrots + 1 tablespoon tahini

Roasted Chickpeas (150 cal)
½ cup

Seaweed Crisps (120 cal)
5 pieces

Sliced Fennel with Lemon and Olive Oil Drizzle (120 cal)
½ cup slices + juice from half a small lemon + 1 tablespoon olive oil

Sliced Zucchini with Avocado Dip (150 cal)
1 cup zucchini sticks + 2 tablespoons mashed avocado

Smoked Salmon on Cucumber Rounds (150 cal)
2 ounces salmon + 6 cucumber slices

Soy Nut Snack Mix (150 cal)
¼ cup

Soy Yogurt with Chia Seeds (150 cal)
¾ cup soy yogurt + 1 tablespoon chia seeds

Spiced Almonds (150 cal)
1 ounce

Steamed Green Beans with Grated Lemon Zest (120 cal)
1 cup green beans with 1 teaspoon zest

Stuffed Medjool Dates (150 cal)
2 dates, each stuffed with ½ teaspoon goat cheese

Stuffed Mini Bell Peppers (150 cal)
2 halves, each stuffed with 1 ounce string cheese

Sunflower Seed Butter on Cucumber Slices (180 cal)
2 tablespoons sunflower seed butter + 6 cucumber slices

Toaster Sweet Potato Slices with Tahini (150 cal)
2 slices + 1 tablespoon tahini

Tofu Cubes with Tamari (100 cal)
½ cup tofu cubes + 2 tablespoons tamari

Tomato and Feta Mini Skewers (150 cal)
3 skewers: 3 cherry tomatoes and 2 small cubes feta each

Trail Mix (No Added Sugar) (150 cal)
¼ cup

Tuna Cucumber Boats (150 cal)
½ cup tuna + 1 cucumber, halved lengthwise and seeded

Turkey Lettuce Wrap Bites (150 cal)
2 slices deli turkey + lettuce

Walnut-Stuffed Figs (150 cal)
2 figs + 1 tablespoon walnuts

Watermelon with Mint (50 cal)
1 cup diced watermelon + fresh mint

Zucchini Rounds with Hummus and Paprika (60 cal)
6 zucchini rounds + 2 tablespoons hummus + paprika

Acknowledgments

First, to my good college friend, Peri Wallace Higgins, who stayed after me and insisted I write the book because it was badly needed and it could help a lot of people. At last, Peri's tenacity won the day. Thank you!

Also, a big thanks to Rachael Ray, who never says no when I ask for something, and who I have worked with for almost twenty years. I couldn't think of anyone better to write these amazing, delicious, fun, accessible recipes that will bring so much joy to so many homes. Your generosity is breathtaking. I love you.

Thanks to my editor, Leah Wilson, who was pitched this idea by my agent and got it right away and immediately wanted to bring my vision to the page and the rest of the world. There's nothing more inspiring than when someone understands, appreciates, and champions your creativity.

Thanks to my agent, Lisa Gallagher, who stands with me in all of my literary endeavors, who never says I can't do something, and who is always there supporting, cheering, and assuring me that it all is very possible. You ride with me so hard and surround me with such positive energy—a fearless, irrepressible teammate that makes me a better and more productive writer, because you're in my corner.

And to my family, Tristé, Dash, and Declan—the home team. The A Team. This is book number thirty. You are the true reason why I have achieved and continue to dream. I love you guys beyond even what my words can aptly describe. Time to go on safari again!

Notes

1. Kenneth Hill, "The Demography of Menopause," *Maturitas* 23 (1996): 113–27, doi.org/10.1016/0378-5122(95)00968-x.
2. Ekta Kapoor, Nancy Safwan, Rajeev Chaudhry, et al., "Addressing Menopause Symptoms: Barriers and Opportunities for Improvement," *Mayo Clinic Proceedings* 100, no. 11 (2025): 1897–07, doi.org/10.1016/j.mayocp.2025.02.018.
3. Ellen W. Freeman, Mary D. Sammel, Hui Lin, et al., "Symptoms Associated with Menopausal Transition and Reproductive Hormones in Midlife Women," pt. 1 *Obstetrics & Gynecology* 110, no. 2 (2007): 230–40, doi.org/10.1097/01.AOG.0000270153.59102.40.
4. Nancy E. Avis, Sybil L. Crawford, Gail Greendale, et al., "Duration of Menopausal Vasomotor Symptoms over the Menopause Transition," *JAMA Internal Medicine* 175, no. 4 (2015): 531–39, doi.org/10.1001/jamainternmed.2014.8063.
5. Sue Thomas, "Genitourinary Syndrome of the Menopause (GSM)," *Urology & Continence Care Today*, Launch Edition, accessed March 2, 2026, www.ucc-today.com/journals/issue/launch-edition/article/genitourinary-syndrome-of-the-menopause-gsm-ucct.
6. Varna Kodoth, Samantha Scaccia, and Brooke Aggarwal, "Adverse Changes in Body Composition During the Menopausal Transition and Relation to Cardiovascular Risk: A Contemporary Review,"

Women's Health Reports 3, no. 1 (2022): 573–81, doi.org/10.1089/whr.2021.0119.

7. Howard M. Kravitz and Hadine Joffe, "Sleep During the Perimenopause: A SWAN Story," *Obstetrics and Gynecology Clinics of North America* 38, no. 3 (2011): 567–86, doi.org/10.1016/j.ogc.2011.06.002.
8. Bone Health & Osteoporosis Foundation, "What Women Need to Know," accessed March 2, 2026, https://www.bonehealthandosteoporosis.org/preventing-fractures/general-facts/what-women-need-to-know.
9. Samar R. El Khoudary, Brooke Aggarwal, Theresa M. Beckie, et al.; American Heart Association Prevention Science Committee of the Council on Epidemiology and Prevention; and Council on Cardiovascular and Stroke Nursing, "Menopause Transition and Cardiovascular Disease Risk: Implications for Timing of Early Prevention: A Scientific Statement from the American Heart Association," *Circulation* 142, no. 25 (2020): e506–32, doi.org/10.1161/CIR.0000000000000912.
10. Taulant Muka, Clare Oliver-Williams, Setor Kunutsor, et al., "Association of Age at Onset of Menopause and Time Since Onset of Menopause with Cardiovascular Outcomes, Intermediate Vascular Traits, and All-Cause Mortality: A Systematic Review and Meta-Analysis," *JAMA Cardiology* 1, no. 7 (2016): 767–76, doi.org/10.1001/jamacardio.2016.2415.
11. Huanquan Liao, Jinping Cheng, Dong Pan, et al., "Association of Earlier Age at Menopause with Risk of Incident Dementia, Brain Structural Indices and the Potential Mediators: A Prospective Community-Based Cohort Study," *eClinicalMedicine* 60 (2023): 102033, doi.org/10.1016/j.eclinm.2023.102033.
12. Megan L. Marsh, Marta Novaes Oliveira, and Victoria J. Vieira-Potter, "Adipocyte Metabolism and Health After the Menopause: The Role of Exercise," *Nutrients* 15, no. 2 (2023): 444, doi.org/10.3390/nu15020444.

13. James Francis Carmody, Sybil Crawford, Elena Salmoirago-Blotcher, et al., "Mindfulness Training for Coping with Hot Flashes: Results of a Randomized Trial," *Menopause* 18, no. 6 (2011): 611–20, doi.org/10.1097/gme.0b013e318204a05c.
14. Michael J. LaMonte, Jean Wactawski-Wende, Joseph C. Larson, et al., "Association of Physical Activity and Fracture Risk Among Postmenopausal Women," *JAMA Network Open* 2, no. 10 (2019): e1914084, doi.org/10.1001/jamanetworkopen.2019.14084.
15. Nancy E. Avis, Alicia Colvin, Joyce T. Bromberger, et al., "Change in Health-Related Quality of Life over the Menopausal Transition in a Multiethnic Cohort of Middle-Aged Women: Study of Women's Health Across the Nation," *Menopause* 16, no. 5 (2009): 860–69, doi.org/10.1097/gme.0b013e3181a3cdaf.
16. Paul M. Ridker, Brendan M. Everett, Tom Thuren, et al., "Anti-Inflammatory Therapy with Canakinumab for Atherosclerotic Disease," *New England Journal of Medicine* 377, no. 12 (2017): 1119–31, doi.org/10.1056/NEJMoa1707914.
17. Samar R. El Khoudary, Xirun Chen, Meiyuzhen Qi, et al., "The Relation Between Systemic Inflammation and the Menopause Transition: The Study of Women's Health Across the Nation," *Journal of Clinical Endocrinology & Metabolism* 110, no. 11 (2025): e3566–76, doi.org/10.1210/clinem/dgaf175.
18. Samara Huckvale, Stephanie Reyes, Alexandra Kulikova, et al., "An Association Between the Inflammatory Biomarker GlycA and Depressive Symptom Severity," *Journal of Clinical Psychiatry* 82, no. 1 (2021): 20m13245, doi.org/10.4088/JCP.20m13245.
19. Tonya Orchard, Vedat Yildiz, Susan E. Steck, et al., "Dietary Inflammatory Index, Bone Mineral Density, and Risk of Fracture in Postmenopausal Women: Results from the Women's Health Initiative," *Journal of Bone and Mineral Research* 32, no. 5 (2017): 1136–46, doi.org/10.1002/jbmr.3070.

20. L. Schwingshackl and G. Hoffmann, "Mediterranean Dietary Pattern, Inflammation and Endothelial Function: A Systematic Review and Meta-Analysis of Intervention Trials," *Nutrition, Metabolism & Cardiovascular Diseases* 24, no. 9 (2014): 929–39. doi.org/10.1016/j.numecd.2014.03.003.
21. Michel Lucas, Geneviève Asselin, Chantal Mérette, et al., "Effects of Ethyl-Eicosapentaenoic Acid Omega-3 Fatty Acid Supplementation on Hot Flashes and Quality of Life Among Middle-Aged Women," *Menopause* 16, no. 2 (2009): 357–66, doi.org/10.1097/gme.0b013e3181865386.
22. Almudena Sánchez-Villegas, Miguel Delgado-Rodríguez, Alvaro Alonso, et al., "Association of the Mediterranean Dietary Pattern with the Incidence of Depression," *Archives of General Psychiatry* 66, no. 10 (2009): 1090–98, doi.org/10.1001/archgenpsychiatry.2009.129.
23. Emily T. Farrell, Michael D. Wirth, Alexander C. McLain, et al., "Associations Between the Dietary Inflammatory Index and Sleep Metrics in the Energy Balance Study (EBS)," *Nutrients* 15, no. 2 (2023): 419, doi.org/10.3390/nu15020419.
24. Larry A. Tucker and Karen Maxwell, "Effects of Weight Training on the Emotional Well-Being and Body Image of Females: Predictors of Greatest Benefit," *American Journal of Health Promotion* 6, no. 5 (1992): 338–44, 371, doi.org/10.4278/0890-1171-6.5.338.

Index

Index

Index

Index

Index

Index

S

Index

Index

S

Index

About the Author

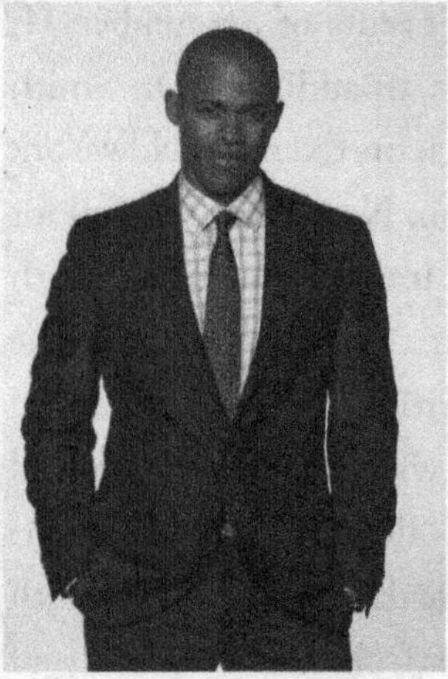

Dr. Ian Smith is the author of thirty books, including the #1 *New York Times* bestselling books *Shred: The Revolutionary Diet*, *Super Shred: The Big Results Diet*, *Blast the Sugar Out!*, *The Clean 20*, *The Ancient Nine*, *Clean & Lean*, and *Fast Burn*, with millions of copies in print. Dr. Smith's Chicago-based detective novels, the Ashe Cayne series, including *The Unspoken*, *Wolf Point*, *The Overnights*, *Eagle Rock*, and *Beyond Midnight*, have been optioned for a television series. His novel *The Ancient Nine*, based on his experiences in one of Harvard's secret societies, has also been optioned for television.

He served as the solo host of the nationally syndicated Emmy award–winning television show *The Doctors* and is a longtime medical contributor to *The Rachael Ray Show*. His podcast, *Conversations with Dr. Ian Smith*, is popular and informative.

He served as the medical/diet expert for six seasons on VH1's highly rated *Celebrity Fit Club*. He is the creator and founder of the national health initiatives The 50 Million Pound Challenge and The Makeover Mile. Dr. Smith is the former medical correspondent for NBC News Network and NewsChannel 4 in New York, where he filed reports for *NBC Nightly News* and *The Today Show*, as well as WNBC's various news broadcasts. He has appeared extensively on numerous broadcasts, including *The Oprah Winfrey Show*, *The View*, *Steve Harvey*, *The Talk*, *Anderson Cooper 360°*, CNN, MSNBC, HLN, and many more. He has written for various publications, including *Time*, *Newsweek*, *Men's Fitness*, and the *New York Daily News*. He has been featured in several other publications, including *People*, *Redbook*, *Details*, *Essence*, *Ebony*, *Cosmopolitan*, and *Black Enterprise*.

A highly sought-after speaker, Dr. Smith's work has been honored by several organizations, including the National Academy of Television Arts & Sciences for his coverage of the momentous events of September 11, 2001. He is also very active in charitable causes. In addition, Dr. Smith has served on the boards of the American Council on Exercise, New York City Mission Society, Prevent Cancer Foundation, New York Council for the Humanities, and Maya Angelou Center for Health Equity. Dr. Smith was honored to be a member of President Obama's health endeavor, the President's Council on Fitness, Sports, and Nutrition.

Dr. Smith graduated from Harvard College with an AB and received a master's in science education from Teachers College of Columbia University. He completed his first two years of medical school at Dartmouth Medical School and earned his medical degree from the University of Chicago Pritzker School of Medicine.

Instagram: @DoctorIanSmith
TikTok: @theofficialDrIan
Facebook: www.facebook.com/Dr.IanKSmith
Website: www.doctoriansmith.com